PRAISE FOR KIMBERLY RAE MILLER'S
BEAUTIFUL BODIES

"Just as she did in *Coming Clean*, Kim writes about pain and struggle with utter honesty, humor, and grace. If you have ever felt at odds with your body—as if no matter what you do, it simply isn't good enough—you will see yourself in this wonderful book. If you have a partner or daughter who struggles with her body, this book is required reading."

—Gabi Moskowitz, producer of Freeform's *Young & Hungry* and co-author of *Hot Mess Kitchen*

"Weaving diet history with all-insecurities-bared personal narrative, Kimberly Rae Miller charts the cuckoo, dangerous, and heartbreaking efforts we endure to suppress our bodies into an imagined ideal. Funny, honest, and deeply empathic, this memoir of the public and private body chronicles the ultimate struggle—not to lose weight but to love the shape of our lives."

—Sarah McColl, founding editor-in-chief of Yahoo Food

"Kimberly Rae Miller's *Beautiful Bodies* will make you laugh and cry with her every-woman story of a life spent chasing a beautiful body. Truthful, heartfelt, and delightfully funny, Miller walks her path toward redemption with admirable grace—and reminds us it's truly okay to be exactly as we are."

—Katie Sise, author of *Creative Girl, The Boyfriend App*, and *The Pretty App*

PRAISE FOR KIMBERLY RAE MILLER'S *COMING CLEAN*

WALL STREET JOURNAL BESTSELLER

AMAZON BEST BOOK OF THE YEAR
IN BIOGRAPHIES AND MEMOIRS

AMAZON BEST BOOK OF THE MONTH

"Reality shows typically stay with hoarders only long enough to portray them as objects of pity or ridicule, but Miller's story, *Coming Clean*, offers a uniquely nuanced look at her intelligent, loving, but broken father and the enduring effect his affliction has had on her and her long-suffering mother."

—*Entertainment Weekly*

"Harrowing. You root for [Kim], you root for [her parents], and at the end, you marvel at the capacity for human resilience."

—*People*

"[Kimberly Rae Miller] recounts a childhood in which it was impossible to shower in her house or cook in the kitchen, of being bitten by fleas and listening to rats rustle at night. The hoarding surrounds everything . . . This searing tale of the damage caused by the disease reflects Miller's deep consideration of her experience; a deeply affecting, remarkably thoughtful, and well-reasoned book, yet the horror is always there. One can only admire Miller's courage in coming clean."

—*Booklist*, Starred Review

"In Kimberly Rae Miller's memoir, *Coming Clean*, the writer doesn't minimize the destruction the disorder causes families. But she uses her own experience to paint a much more compassionate and nuanced portrait of the illness than is usually shown on reality TV shows like *Hoarders*."

—*The Associated Press*

"As a child Miller realized her family wasn't like other people's families with tidy, presentable homes; far from it. Miller never invited anyone home and had to adopt a 'decoy' house to be dropped off at by friends . . . Stuff and unused purchases were piled so high that little room was left for the family even to eat or sleep or use the bathrooms."

—*Publishers Weekly*

"[An] honest, sensitive memoir . . . At the heart of *Coming Clean* lie two equally mysterious phenomena, one as timely as the other is timeless. Hoarding, the first, has only recently entered the popular lexicon while the second, familial love, spans the ages."

—*Washington Independent Review of Books*

"Miller renders her harrowing account without self-pity, and her empathy for her parents, as well as her refusal to treat the hoarding as a spectacle, allow space for redemption—both theirs and her own."

—*Elle*

"Kimberly Rae Miller writes with insight about growing up the daughter of a hoarder in her family's moldy, flea-infested home—and eventually overcoming her anger and shame."

—*Parade*

"An engrossing, sympathetic exploration of living with hoarder parents."

—*Kirkus Reviews*

"Astonishingly honest and heartfelt . . . Kimberly Rae Miller's new memoir comes clean on how the reality of compulsive hoarding is very different from what we see on TV."

—*The Daily Beast*, Women in the World

"*Coming Clean* is shocking and painful, but it's also full of warmth and compassion . . . in some ways a tribute to Miller's deeply imperfect parents."

—*PureWow*

"Miller's wry retelling of her upbringing will encourage others who also did not emerge from the cookie cutter."

—*Library Journal*

"Kimberly Rae Miller is a brave and gifted writer, and her insightful examination of her troubled relationship with her parents will speak to anyone who has ever struggled to hide a family secret. *Coming Clean* is a standout coming-of-age memoir. A must read."

—Kjerstin Gruys, author of *Mirror, Mirror Off the Wall*

"Turn off the reality TV and read *Coming Clean*, an engrossing, beautifully written memoir of growing up in a hoarding family that treats its subject with humanity and grace."

—Doreen Orion, author of *Queen of the Road*

Beautiful Bodies

ALSO BY KIMBERLY RAE MILLER

Coming Clean

Beautiful Bodies

a memoir

Kimberly Rae Miller

Little
a

Published by Little A, New York

www.apub.com

Amazon, the Amazon logo, and Little A are trademarks of Amazon.com, Inc., or its affiliates.

ISBN-13: 9781503935174 (hardcover)
ISBN-10: 1503935175 (hardcover)

ISBN-13: 9781477829578 (paperback)
ISBN-10: 1477829571 (paperback)

Cover design by Rachel Adam Rogers

Printed in the United States of America

First edition

For Roy, my Superman

PATIENCE AND FORTITUDE

The first time I walked into the New York Public Library, I took one look around and walked right back out. It's an intimidating place: an enormous marble Beaux Arts beast of a building, with mazes of stairwells and dark wood shelves filled with thousands of books you're not allowed to touch. And lions guard it. Colossal marble lions named Patience and Fortitude.

I will need patience and fortitude if I am going to find the answers I need. Answers to dull the constant, anxious stress of obsession.

What is the ideal human body?

Why don't we all have it? Why do we come in different shapes and sizes, and when and why did we start hating ourselves for it?

Simple stuff.

I wake up every morning and go to work with brilliant people who have done brilliant things. They've run magazines and published books, merged companies and built empires, and they trust me to edit diet books for celebrities and gurus who want nothing more than to impart their wisdom to the strangers who love them (or will as soon as they finish their book). Between books I write blogs without bylines for a variety of health experts and websites: articles about the opiate qualities of lettuce and how kale is miraculous in its superfoodiness (but might also destroy your thyroid) and which nondairy milk is the best nondairy milk for bikini season. Throughout the day I take pictures of the food I'm eating so that I can write about it later on my own blog, where I try to undo some of the damage I may have caused between the hours of nine and six by reminding the small group of people who follow my digital life (and myself, mostly) that health isn't defined by a pant size.

My favorite part of each day happens before I dole out a single word of anonymous advice. It happens while I sip my first cup of artificially sweetened coffee and roll my feet over a spiky stress ball I was gifted at a press event for spiky-stress-ball yoga. It comes in the form of a barrage of press releases about guaranteed weight loss and breaking studies that find their way into my inbox overnight and have been sitting in wait for me to add them to my to-do list. Most of them are nonsense; experts no one has ever heard of promising results that defy the laws of physics. But every once in a while there will be something I haven't seen before, something that makes sense, something backed by numbers and data, research done by people far more educated than I am. Every morning I open my email in hopes of finding some previously unknown nugget of truth that will save ~~me~~ us all from being on the wrong end of some malefic statistic. And by the end of the workday, I will have a new diet to fall in love with.

My career was a complete accident, but it was always in the making: I'm addicted to dieting. I've never met a diet I didn't want to try. Okay, maybe the Master Cleanse (I imagine there's a lot of heartburn involved), but other than that I would try them all, and I have. Well, most of them. I have eaten nothing but meat, nothing but raw vegetables, nothing but fruit, nothing but juice. I have counted points, calories, and macros; scarfed down all my meals in a six-hour feeding window; banished gluten and dairy; and had preportioned food delivered to my apartment in the wee hours of the morning by elves. I have paid an arthritic old Romanian woman in a dentist's office to sodomize me with a hose, flood my colon with filtered water, and then suck my feces out with that very same hose. All of it in the name of weight loss. Dieting is my only real hobby.

I have come to rely on the structure and hope diets provide as a way of anchoring myself in the world. When there are no rules or promises to life, a diet provides them. When things are at their most stressful, calorie counting is a refuge of control. I am aware that this is very much in line with disordered eating behavior. I have no concept of what *ordered* eating behavior looks like. I'm not in the slightest bit alone, though: disordered eating has become so culturally ubiquitous that we now have a name for people who are too healthy, relentlessly healthy, people who take every article someone like me writes to heart and adjust their life accordingly. Orthorexia is just one of a long list of new feeding and eating disorders we can now be classified as having. I don't know many people who don't agonize about every meal, whether to leave the table proud but unfulfilled or guilt riddled but sated. Or those who have spent so long having that fight that they have given up completely, defeated, resolved to punish themselves indefinitely for being hungry, as if eating were the most depraved thing they could choose to do with their time. Culturally, we seem to have lost the ability to exist in the in-between. In a country where children are bombarded with junk-food advertising between cartoons[1] and then consistently berated for their lack of health or aesthetic as they age into adulthood, it is hardly surprising.

And I am a hypocrite, because while I spend my days doling out diet advice from the safe anonymity of my computer screen, I know that diets are in many ways a fantasy: studies have consistently shown that long-term dieting doesn't work and that the number-one predictor

---

1. Nearly 70 percent of commercials on Nickelodeon are for junk food, which is reduced quite a bit from the 2005 level of almost 90 percent. Adults fare better, with only 20 percent of their advertising being for unhealthy food—but that's still a significant amount.

of future weight gain is prior dieting. People can, on average, lose 10 to 15 percent of their body weight easily and successfully with just about any diet that restricts calories through one ploy or another, but in time 97 percent will gain it back with interest, leaving them in worse health than they would have been in if they had just not dieted to begin with.

The weight-loss industry is worth $60 billion a year—and about $60,000 of that is my fault. Delivered by brave and beautiful heroes sporting spandex on morning shows and middle-of-the-night infomercials, diets are sold as altruism, but they are rooted in shame.

They need to be. They wouldn't be profitable if they weren't. If we stopped being ashamed of our bodies, the whole diet industry would collapse. I like being employed, so I have mixed feelings about that, but I could probably find another job, and I would be curious to see a society that doesn't revolve around people constantly trying to hate themselves into perfection.

Which is why I am once again standing in front of the New York City Public Library, willing myself to go inside and get some answers about this cultural obsession I've made a career out of. There's a librarian named Richard waiting for me.

After my panic attack in the lobby a few weeks earlier, I decided it was best to ask for help. When in doubt, find someone with a master's degree who knows what they're doing. It took about a week between sending my plea for research help into the vast unknown of the New York Public Library's "Contact Us" page and getting an invitation from Richard to come in and sit down with him to talk about my research project.

There was a time, a long time ago, when I knew how to rock a library. My family moved to a new town when I was seven. Our house had burned down in an electrical fire, not a particularly rare occurrence thanks to the shoddy wiring common in the small ticky-tacky-style houses endemic to the south shore of Long Island, a product of the post–World War II mass housing production. There were three other fires in our district that night; in one of them a two-year-old boy had died. And so we never complained about having to rebuild our life—it could have been worse. My mother reminded us every day that in the end, life could always get worse. And so we set about finding all new everything like it was an adventure: new clothes, new furniture, new dogs, new friends, and new library cards. Our first stop after moving what few items we'd cobbled together in our hotel into our new house was the library. While my mother waited for furniture to be delivered, my father and I drove to Main Street to introduce ourselves to our new library.

It was only a matter of months before my dad knew all the staff by name, and they would chide him for only returning a portion of the books he took out each week. The scolding was real, but the angry faces were not. My father is charming, a jolly absentminded-professor type, minus actual academia, and even the sternest of the bunch would soften after he confessed that he loved those books so much he couldn't bear to bring them back.[2] More likely than not they were lost to the piles of newspapers, books, and magazines my father constantly surrounded himself with in his search for answers on just about everything.

He signed me up for the children's newspaper club—against my will—in what I suspect was an attempt to keep me occupied after school so he could browse the shelves in peace for an hour or two without my constant begging for a dollar for the Italian ice cart strategically stationed outside. It was there, in newspaper club, that I landed my first and only cover story in an award-winning exposé about racism in our town. That's a lie; in reality I wrote three hundred words about why racism is bad. I can tell you now that it was a biased piece, as I was my only source and I neglected to do any real research into the opposing proracism stance. I'm pretty sure my dad was the only one who read it. He assured me it was excellent.

---

2.   I'm relatively sure my college fund was spent on library fees.

It wasn't long before our hometown library became a refuge, babysitter, entertainer, soothsayer, and therapist. If I was grappling with something I didn't understand—hormones, homework, boys, or bullies—I would find a book by someone who did understand, and the world seemed a lot more manageable.

And then the Internet happened. Now I mostly use my library card to take out a few of my less estimable literary indulgences, not wanting my bookshelves at home to serve as evidence of my love for sexy were-wolves and quirky New Jersey bounty hunters. So it was natural that the Internet was my first stop when I started to harp on the idea of the ideal body, what it meant, and why we were all so obsessed with having one. But the Internet failed me; all I could find were fluff pieces about how Marilyn Monroe was a size twelve (she wasn't[3]) and how history had once revered a fatter physique as a sign of wealth and posterity (not as true as we seem to think).

I was surprisingly nervous standing in front of the research desk, waiting for my blind date with Richard the Librarian, looking around every few seconds while I straightened the book-request forms and organized their pencils so that they all faced downward—so as not to inadvertently stab someone. If the research staff minded me cleaning up their workspace, they didn't let on. I clean when I'm nervous. And I was nervous that this keeper of intellectual pursuits would see right through my research request and know that I was on the verge of giving up dieting forever—and with it any professional integrity I had.

I'd been on a diet for over twenty years; two-thirds of my life had been spent thinking about food and how to avoid it, and I was tired of

---

3.   Marilyn Monroe probably measured around a size four in today's sizing, with a bit of tailoring needed to bring in the waist. She had a very dramatic hourglass figure, with a twenty-two-inch waist and thirty-five-inch hips, and a bra size of 36D. Her dressmaker records her weight as being 118 pounds and her height five foot four and a half inches.

analyzing every sandwich I met. But I didn't know how to eat without a diet. I didn't know what my body was supposed to look like or how to see it as anything more than a "before" photo.

"Ms. Miller?" Richard did not look like I expected him to. I expected a sexy-geeky grad student, with tousled hair and square-framed glasses—I'd cast him as a young John Cusack in the movie in my mind. But Richard looked more like Al Bundy.

"Hi." I gave him my best pageant smile. It's possible that I curtseyed.

"Follow me," he said, leading me to an enclosed glass cubicle in the middle of one of the study rooms, with a single desk and computer.

An arm's-length booklist about the history of beauty was already waiting for me on his desk. Corsets, lead-laden makeup, and foot binding seemed to be well-documented elements of human history, but as I browsed the resources he'd clearly painstakingly gathered, I couldn't find a single book that was capable of telling me what the objective, scientific, quantifiable ideal of a beautiful body is, or what we've done in search of it.

"This isn't exactly what I was looking for," I said. "Can you show me how to search the articles and journals database?" I asked.

"What exactly are you looking for, Ms. Miller?"

———

Before smartphones, before (almost) all the answers were on the Internet, I started to carry a little book with me everywhere I went: a tiny worn encyclopedia of foods and their corresponding calories. It went with me to sleepovers and on school field trips, and I wrote down every single thing that entered my mouth in a notebook I stole from my father. I didn't know how much I should eat, but I knew less was better, and each day I had a competition with myself to eat less than the day before.

In seventh grade I was called to the school counselors' office because another student had reported me for having disordered-eating behavior.

It was the nineties; heroin chic was in and eating disorders seemed to be a rite of passage. One of the counselors handed me a few pamphlets about proper nutrition and self-esteem and called my mother.

"Does my daughter look like she's starving?" she asked.

I didn't, he agreed, and he sent me back to class. I was failing at anorexia, but hey, at least somebody had noticed I was trying.

By high school, a lunch period was no longer required, and I feigned academic overeagerness so that I could schedule an extra class in lieu of eating. Every day of grades ten through twelve, I had two white-cheddar rice cakes as my midday meal between third and fourth period. By the time school was over, I would be starving, and I would more often than not end up binging on whatever I could find at home or at a nearby fast-food restaurant. Sometimes I would throw it up; sometimes I wouldn't—I far preferred not eating at all to vomiting.

At college night in my junior year, I signed up to be recruited for the Navy. Not because of a deep-seated interest in serving my country, but because I thought boot camp might be a good weight-loss opportunity. I was turned down because I have asthma, but my parents still get calls from recruiters asking if I'd be interested in a career in the military.

While working as an actress in my early twenties, my weight became a commodity to be hired and fired by. I would get calls from my agent requesting current measurements on a bimonthly basis because my weight seemed to fluctuate constantly. Despite my constant obsessing, I was never particularly thin.

I could maintain a size eight, but it took herculean effort, near starvation, and a religious gym routine that often left little time for actual acting.

By twenty-five I had become a grizzled industry vet and decided it might be time to consider giving up acting. The truth was, I had just gone through a bad breakup and put on about thirty pounds. (Putting on a large amount of weight in a short period of time is one of my specialties.)

I didn't want to show up to auditions looking the way I did, so I applied to law school—it seemed like a logical progression at the time.

Before I could decide, I saw a casting notice that I had to submit for. It was for an online talk show for a magazine-publishing company. I ended up hosting a little web series called *The Daily Special* and later an online scripted episodic called *Pretty Imperfect*, both on a site called Elastic Waist: A Growing Obsession with the Weight of It All. The show would eventually lead to a writing career, at first for the Condé Nast blog network and then for other fitness-related websites and news outlets. In the irony of all ironies, my lifelong struggle between dieting constantly and finding peace with my body had led to a career I loved. I had my own little space in the world where I could talk about being a "normal" girl, someone who always seemed to have anywhere between five and thirty real or imagined pounds to lose. But everything I wrote was with one very specific message: Love yourself anyway. You don't have to be a size two to be beautiful. Life's too short to never eat cake.

It was, and is, a great message. I just didn't believe it when it came to my own body.

I've heard of a mythical tribe of people who love their bodies, who never fret over the size of stomachs or thighs, their body-fat percentage, or whether they can "get away with" wearing whatever the newest "in" thing to wear is. Those people are unicorns and they should be treasured, because they haven't let society totally screw them up. That is, if they really exist.

So with all of this history behind me, when Richard the Librarian asked what I was looking for, I knew I was looking for a reason. A reason I couldn't be happy with any of my accomplishments if I was over a size eight. I'd done real, tangible things I could be proud of, should be proud of, in my life. But if my size didn't match my success level, it was moot. I'm not alone, because if I were, I'd be out of a job, so I wanted to know why *we* are like this. I was hoping there was a book that Richard could find me that would explain it all.

ONE

THE INUIT DIET

Vilhjalmur Stefansson was a real-life parka-wearing Indiana Jones,[1] a man of two worlds. An Arctic explorer, he spent years at a time living among the Inuit in the Arctic Archipelago, learning their language, hunting among them, and even marrying and having a child with an Inuit woman, Fannie Pannigabluk.[2] He was also a New York socialite and a tad bit of a playboy who captivated public interest; when he wasn't exploring the most brutal parts of Canada, Stefansson enjoyed celebrity status as a bestselling author and lecturer.

He was also an inadvertent diet guru. While his coterie of colleagues often embarked upon their Arctic journeys with boats full of Western dietary staples—flour, canned meats, and vegetables meant to

---

1. Stefansson actually appeared as a character in *Indiana Jones and the Philosopher's Stone* by Max McCoy, a 1995 novel based on the George Lucas films. In the story, Stefansson is a haughty New York anthropologist, intent on keeping Indiana out of the prestigious Explorers Club, which Stefansson was actually president of between 1919 and 1922, not 1933 when the book is set.

2. Whom he later abandoned but continued to support financially. While Stefansson continued to date a number of high-profile women in New York, he waited until after Pannigabluk died in 1940, when he was sixty-one, to remarry, to the twenty-eight-year-old singer and actress Evelyn Schwartz Baird.

ward off malnutrition—Stefansson considered his full immersion into Inuit culture a chance to study the effects of a high-fat, high-protein, low-carbohydrate diet on health and dental hygiene. Using himself as a guinea pig, Stefansson subsisted on the same seal, walrus, fish, and whale meat his Inuit hosts did, and according to him, his health thrived.

Stefansson's diet stalwartly contradicted the low-fat, high-carbohydrate, calorie-obsessed culture that dominated the 1920s, thanks to the first-ever calorie-counting manual published in 1918 by Dr. Lulu Hunt Peters, the Susan Powter[3] of her day, a no-nonsense diet sage who had struggled with obesity throughout her life. She offered herself as an example of the willpower and determination necessary for thinness and warned against consuming more than 1,200 calories a day in her bestselling diet guide *Diet and Health: With Key to the Calories*. While Hunt's diet book has long since been usurped on the bestseller list,[4] her 1,200-calorie-a-day guideline has remained a staple of low-calorie diets in the ninety years since its publishing.

In 1928, backed by a grant by the Institute of American Meat Packers, Stefansson and fellow Arctic explorer Karsten Anderson embarked on a year-long study—using only themselves as the test group and the general population as the inadvertent control—to prove that a meat-centric diet, consisting of high protein and fat, was sufficient in providing the human body with all the essential nutrients it needed for survival, including vitamin C, a vital nutrient that the human body cannot produce on its own and that is most readily obtained through fruits and vegetables. With medical supervision by Dr. Eugene DuBois and his team at Bellevue Hospital in New York City, the duo undertook a yearlong menu of fish, chops, organ meats, bone marrow, and broth, coffee, and tea. At the end of the year, both men were in almost

---

3.   "Stop the Insanity!"
4.   *Diet and Health: With Key to the Calories* is still available for purchase on Amazon.com.

exactly the same shape they'd started in. Each lost a negligible amount of weight, neither suffered from scurvy brought on by a vitamin C deficiency, and Stefansson even ended the experiment with better dental health than he'd started with. The outcome was exactly what Stefansson had hypothesized: human beings can survive on meat and meat alone, and he went on to write about his Inuit diet in *Harper's Bazaar* and later in his books *Not by Bread Alone* (1946) and *The Fat of the Land* (1956). And while Stefansson never set out to prove that the Inuit were a lean, six-pack-donning society, low-carb-diet gurus would quote his yearlong experiment for decades as historical evidence that meat is the secret to an ideal body.

My first attempt at following the Inuit diet took place in 1987.

I was four.

I didn't know who Vilhjalmur Stefansson was, and I probably wouldn't have been able to point out Canada on a map, but I knew about the Inuit people thanks to *Sesame Street*. While I enjoyed a good life-lesson-bestowing puppet as much as any preschooler, my favorite *Sesame Street* segments were the five-minute documentaries that featured kids my age, living lives infinitely more interesting than my own.

In this thirty-year-old memory, I watch as the *Sesame Street* crew follows an Inuit girl living in Arctic Alaska as she goes about her daily life. She spends a little time with her grandfather in a hut he'd made from snow (a real-life igloo) that he'd use while fishing and helps her mother prepare food in their perfectly status quo (read: non-igloo) house. From what I could tell, life revolved mostly around not freezing to death. Her key to survival: eating fat. She said something along the lines of "We eat fat to stay warm in the winter." And that was all it took. My first piece of diet advice.

I looked at my father, who seemed to be enthralled by the old man in the igloo, for some sort of recognition that he too understood the life change we needed to make.

Long Island gets cold in the winter. Not Arctic-survival cold, but unpleasantly chilly. After the Inuit girl waved goodbye and Guy Smiley was back hosting a game show, I was on a mission: a mission to eat as much fat as possible and never be cold again.

Each night while my mother prepared dinner, I would stand in the doorway of the kitchen, asking questions and feigning interest in her day. I had one goal, though: to snatch each soft, creamy globule of fat that she'd carefully trimmed from the steak, pork chop, or chicken she'd prepared as soon as it hit the cutting board. She would tell me about her day with "Grandma Bernice," a lady she worked with whose son, Kim, had played bass for Isaac Hayes and died shortly before I was born from complications from obesity—I was named after him. Whenever she would turn around to wash her hands or throw something away, I would snatch a piece of fat from the counter and shovel it into my mouth before she turned around, rushing to swallow before she could see that I was chewing something and ask me what it was. I never stole all the fat in fear of being discovered; I just took the juiciest-looking pieces.

Once I had a taste for fat, its creamy, savory essence that evolved into a chewy, salty gum of sorts, I knew that the Inuit were onto something. Fat is delicious. And it would keep me warm. Food had a purpose. I realized that what I ate could have an effect on my life, on my overall happiness. I'd never given much thought to my body—it was just my body—but now it was something I could control . . . with food.

YOU SHOULD
BE ASHAMED OF
YOURSELF

We can trace our body-shaming ways back to the Bible. Right there, *in the beginning*, Adam and Eve just hung out in the Garden of Eden, being naked and loving it: "And they were both naked, the man and his wife, and were not ashamed."

Their shameless, naked unemployment lasts for only a few paragraphs. Once they eat something that they aren't supposed to,[1] everything changes: their bodies become totems of ignominy, and they are left scrambling to sew a few fig leaves together to cover themselves, to

---

1. Even the food at the heart of our biblical fall from grace is mired in controversy. While the forbidden fruit is often depicted as an apple, a fig, or a pomegranate, some religious scholars believe the forbidden fruit in the Garden of Eden was wheat. In this alternative telling, the wheat in the Garden grew on trees in the form of fully baked bread, and only after Adam and Eve's disobedience was it relegated as punishment to be grown in the ground and refined through manual labor. Carbs, the original sin.

hide their bodies. Our human history is littered with shamed bodies, whether it be based on weight, complexion, foot size, the length of skirts and height of necklines, or any number of deemed inadequacies we have decided upon. What remains constant is that somewhere along the way, being ashamed of one's body became the proper thing to do.

The Bible was inspiration for America's first diet-reform movement, led by none other than cracker namesake Rev. Sylvester Graham. The graham cracker was invented in 1829, not as a vehicle for chocolate and marshmallows but as a way to ward off unholy sexual urges through good old-fashioned wheat germ. Graham, a Presbyterian minister, became America's first diet guru in the early 1830s when he toured the country, preaching his nutritive gospel. He warned that diet, health, and morality were inseparable, and in order to maintain balance between the three, spices, tea, coffee, refined grains, milk, meat, alcohol, and tobacco should be avoided entirely. In fact, the only way to ensure foods did not excite the spirit and lead to depravity was to follow a simple diet of vegetables, unrefined flour, and clean water. In other words, boringness is next to godliness.

So afraid of masturbation was the American public—a topic Graham acutely focused on in his lectures about moral dietary obligation—that Graham's sparse vegetarian diet became a craze of sorts. The lean, hallowed look of his followers became a telltale sign of their piety, and Grahamite boarding houses started appearing all over the country so that his bread-and-vegetable-eating brethren could live with one another outside temptation's grasp. For those Grahamites who had families and homes of their own, specialty supply stores run for and by his disciples opened so that they could do their shopping without fear of provocation. College campuses such as Oberlin, Wesleyan, and Williams opened Grahamite cafeterias for students and staff to frequent without fear of exposure to immoral foods. *The Graham Journal of Health and Longevity*, the country's first health magazine, became a preeminent source for nutrition information in Jacksonian America.

Graham died in 1851 at the ripe old age of fifty-seven, his death disillusioning many of his followers who believed that following his strict plan would not only guarantee them a place in heaven but would ensure a long, healthy life. Despite his early demise[2] there were still many who remained faithful to his dietary teachings. Graham's gospel lived on in the home of John Preston and Ann Janette Stanley Kellogg, devout Christians who raised their sons Will Keith and John Harvey on Graham's principles. Shortly after his graduation from New York University Medical College at Bellevue Hospital in 1875, John Harvey Kellogg took a position as chief physician at the Western Health Reform Institute in Battle Creek, Michigan, a health resort founded on the teachings of the Seventh-day Adventist Church. The teachings mirrored those of Graham's when it came to the relationship between food and morality. Shortly after his arrival, Kellogg renamed the institute the Battle Creek Sanitarium, and while it may have sounded like a hospital, clientele were rarely sick and always well off.

Kellogg's dedication to the diet and morality lessons of his childhood would become a guiding principle behind his work at "The San," where he regularly lectured on the dangers of tea and bouillon consumption among the faithful. Kellogg remained dedicated to the idea that a diet full of whole grains and unprocessed foods and bereft of spices, caffeine, and alcohol would alleviate ungodly sexual urges and serve as a cure for masturbation and premarital sex. Kellogg was so committed to his belief that "sex breeds evil diseases" that he never consummated his marriage to his wife of forty-one years, Ella Eaton. However, he was relatively svelte.

---

2. Actually, not so early. A census of mortality from 1850 found that the average white American had a life expectancy of between 38.3 and 44.0 years of age—experts today believe that those numbers are slightly skewed because deaths were unevenly registered and because the census was taken during cholera and smallpox epidemics.

It was while experimenting with Graham-approved ingredients to create a breakfast cereal worthy of the steep price tag of a stay at The San that Kellogg created corn flakes.[3] But it was his far less religious brother, Will Keith Kellogg, who made them a household name (and himself a very wealthy man) by adding sugar.

---

3. Kellogg was often found tinkering in The San's kitchen, where he is said to have invented eighty grain- and nut-based products, including peanut butter. The Kellogg brothers patented their peanut butter–making process in 1895 and, according to the National Peanut Board, marketed it as a protein source suitable for the dentally impaired.

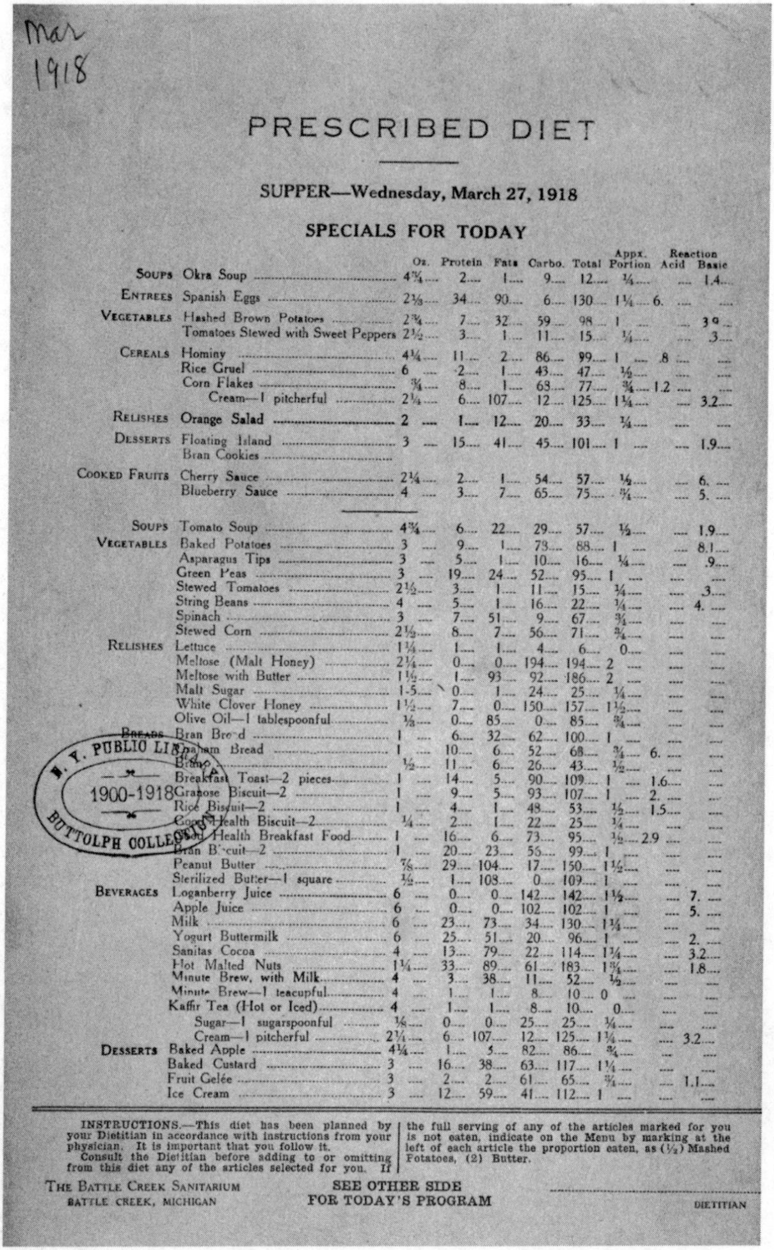

Mar 1918

PRESCRIBED DIET

SUPPER—Wednesday, March 27, 1918

SPECIALS FOR TODAY

		Oz.	Protein	Fats	Carbo.	Total	Appx. Portion	Reaction Acid	Reaction Basic
Soups	Okra Soup	4¾	2	1	9	12	¼		1.4
Entrees	Spanish Eggs	2⅓	34	90	6	130	1¼	6.	
Vegetables	Hashed Brown Potatoes	2¾	7	32	59	98	1		3.9
	Tomatoes Stewed with Sweet Peppers	2½	3	1	11	15	¼		.3
Cereals	Hominy	4¼	11	2	86	99	1	.8	
	Rice Gruel	6	2	1	43	47	½		
	Corn Flakes	¾	8	1	68	77	¾	1.2	
	Cream—1 pitcherful	2¼	6	107	12	125	1¼		3.2
Relishes	Orange Salad	2	1	12	20	33	¼		
Desserts	Floating Island	3	15	41	45	101	1		1.9
	Bran Cookies								
Cooked Fruits	Cherry Sauce	2¼	2	1	54	57	½		6.
	Blueberry Sauce	4	3	7	65	75	¾		5.
Soups	Tomato Soup	4¾	6	22	29	57	½		1.9
Vegetables	Baked Potatoes	3	9	1	78	88	1		8.1
	Asparagus Tips	3	5	1	10	16	¼		.9
	Green Peas	3	19	24	52	95	1		
	Stewed Tomatoes	2½	3	1	11	15	¼		.3
	String Beans	4	5	1	16	22	¼		4.
	Spinach	3	7	51	9	67	¾		
	Stewed Corn	2½	8	7	56	71	¾		
Relishes	Lettuce	1¼	1	1	4	6	0		
	Meltose (Malt Honey)	2¼	0	0	194	194	2		
	Meltose with Butter	1½	1	93	92	186	2		
	Malt Sugar	1-5	0	1	24	25	¼		
	White Clover Honey	1½	7	0	150	157	1½		
	Olive Oil—1 tablespoonful	⅓	0	85	0	85	¾		
Breads	Bran Bread	1	6	32	62	100	1		
	Graham Bread	1	10	6	52	68	¾	6.	
	Bran[illegible]	½	11	6	26	43	½		
	Breakfast Toast—2 pieces	1	14	5	90	109	1	1.6	
	Granose Biscuit—2	1	9	5	93	107	1	2.	
	Rice Biscuit—2	1	4	1	48	53	½	1.5	
	Good Health Biscuit—2	¼	2	1	22	25	¼		
	Good Health Breakfast Food	1	16	6	73	95	½	2.9	
	Bran Biscuit—2	1	20	23	56	99	1		
	Peanut Butter	⅞	29	104	17	150	1½		
	Sterilized Butter—1 square	½	1	108	0	109	1		
Beverages	Loganberry Juice	6	0	0	142	142	1½		7.
	Apple Juice	6	0	0	102	102	1		5.
	Milk	6	23	73	34	130	1¼		
	Yogurt Buttermilk	6	25	51	20	96	1		2.
	Sanitas Cocoa	4	13	79	22	114	1¼		3.2
	Hot Malted Nuts	1¼	33	89	61	183	1¾		1.8
	Minute Brew, with Milk	4	3	38	11	52	½		
	Minute Brew—1 teacupful	4	1	1	8	10	0		
	Kaffir Tea (Hot or Iced)	4	1	1	8	10	0		
	Sugar—1 sugarspoonful	⅛	0	0	25	25	¼		
	Cream—1 pitcherful	2¼	6	107	12	125	1¼		3.2
Desserts	Baked Apple	4¼	1	5	82	86	¾		
	Baked Custard	3	16	38	63	117	1¼		
	Fruit Gelée	3	2	2	61	65	¾		1.1
	Ice Cream	3	12	59	41	112	1		

INSTRUCTIONS.—This diet has been planned by your Dietitian in accordance with instructions from your physician. It is important that you follow it.

Consult the Dietitian before adding to or omitting from this diet any of the articles selected for you. If the full serving of any of the articles marked for you is not eaten, indicate on the Menu by marking at the left of each article the proportion eaten, as (½) Mashed Potatoes, (2) Butter.

The Battle Creek Sanitarium
Battle Creek, Michigan

SEE OTHER SIDE FOR TODAY'S PROGRAM

DIETITIAN

1818 menu from the Battle Creek Sanitarium.

BATTLE CREEK SANITARIUM

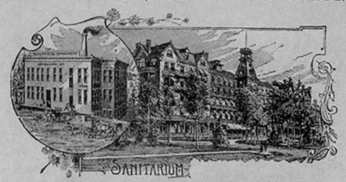

HEALTH FOODS

The line of health foods manufactured by the **SANITARIUM HEALTH FOOD CO.** is so well and favorably known, that little needs to be said as to their quality and genuineness.

The demand for these foods originated at the Battle Creek Sanitarium, itself a pioneer in reforms, where was felt the necessity of providing suitable dietetic preparations of a special character.

The standard raised at the inception of the enterprise has been maintained and elevated by scrupulous attention to details and the utilization of the unequaled facilities afforded by the extensive laboratories of the Sanitarium; hence, all foods produced by this company can be relied upon as being

STRICTLY PURE, and Made with Special Reference to Healthful Properties, rather than to command a sale. Prominent among the different foods may be mentioned

Granola, highly nutritious and toothsome. The process of preparation is such that every element of an irritating character is eliminated. Thoroughly cooked and **READY FOR USE.** One pound more than equals three pounds of best beef in nutrient value.

Granose. A NEW CEREAL FOOD, thoroughly sterilized. Its use clears the tongue and stomach of germs. **CURES** constipation, biliousness, sick-headache, and indigestion. A capital food for sedentary people. Good for everybody, both sick and well.

GRANOSE is the invention of a physician of many years' experience. GRANOLA received highest award at the Columbian and Atlanta Expositions, and GRANOSE a special gold medal at the latter.

For circular describing complete line of Health Foods address,

BATTLE CREEK SANITARIUM HEALTH FOOD CO.,
Battle Creek, Mich.

List of Battle Creek Sanitarium health foods.

———

I remember the exact moment I started to see myself as nothing but a failed body. I was in second grade and I weighed 125 pounds.

I didn't actually. I just thought I did. My mother weighed 125 pounds. She had mentioned her weight in passing and I, not being great with pronouns or active listening, decided she was talking about me. I didn't know how much I was supposed to weigh at seven, but I knew that 125 pounds was too much—I could tell by her tone. I wasn't overweight, but I wasn't skinny and knobby kneed either; I was tall and broad and sturdy, and by second grade I was already sharing shoes with my mom. I was just your average second grader totting around elementary school in size seven white leather pumps. Doctors and relatives and people in the grocery store told me that I was "big for my age," which I took as a compliment; taking up more space than other children whether in pounds or inches (or shoe sizes) seemed to mean I was winning an unspoken contest against my peers.

Up until that point in my childhood, "fat" was a word solely used to describe meat trimmings. It hadn't even occurred to me that a person could be fat. For me every pound gained had been considered a triumph. But something in my mother's tone when she said the words "one twenty-five" made it clear to me that there were rules to body size, and I was inadvertently breaking them. Being "bigger" was most definitely not better, and in that moment something changed in the way I felt about my body—about myself. My body was no longer an extension of my thoughts or feelings, but something else entirely: a betrayer. I allowed these new feelings of sadness and failure to consume me, for hours, maybe a day, before I finally broke under the weight of my despair and started to cry in the middle of quiet study at school.

My mother and I had recently left Long Island—and my father— behind to take care of my sick grandmother in the Bronx. As a whole I far preferred public school in the city to my uniformed private school back home: the kids were nicer. The teachers were another story. Compared to my teachers at home, who had been kind and coddling and put stickers on all my schoolwork, my new teacher, an older woman, ironically named Ms. Weight, didn't fawn over any of us or our nascent brilliance, and therefore I'd resolved that she didn't seem to like children very much. I'm sure she wouldn't have taken kindly to my dramatics, but as luck would have it she had stepped out of the classroom, probably for a smoke break, when my breakdown occurred. In her absence I had an audience of astonishingly sympathetic seven- and eight-year-olds to console me as I mumbled about my weight through my tears. One boy in my class whom I remember in caricature, a prototypical chubby prankster with a repertoire of snarky one-liners and a heart of gold and a Kid 'n Play haircut because it was 1990, assured me I didn't weigh 125. He weighed ninety pounds, he told me confidently, and was sure I was smaller than he was. And with a smile he told me that even if I was 125 pounds, who cared? I could sit next to him and we could just not care together.

Just not caring wasn't an option. Not for me.

When I came home from school, I shared my self-loathing with my mother, who laughed at me and pulled out a pink time-bleached scale from the bathroom of my grandmother's apartment: I weighed sixty pounds, maybe a few pounds more or less, but I remember thinking I weighed almost half of what my mother did, what I thought I did. I stood corrected, but those feelings of utter disappointment in my body, and myself, once kindled, never ceased. In the few short hours I was 125 pounds, I had realized something very important: there was no room for fat in my life. Every snack commercial boasting its "fat-free" status I saw between TV shows, every weight-loss ad featuring a skinny woman wearing enormous pants—showing off her newly smaller, newly better body—seemed to be speaking directly to me. The message was loud and clear: fat is bad. From that moment on I was at war with my body. Suddenly, my goal was to take up as little space in the world as possible, and it would become my lifelong mission to figure out the best way to do just that.

A short while later my mother ordered herself a set of Tony Little exercise VHS tapes from the Home Shopping Network. They promised to whittle away problem areas, and as far as I was concerned, every area of my seven-year-old body was a problem. I quickly claimed them as my own, and each night after dinner I religiously marched in place, crunched, kicked, and flexed in front of the television while my mother and grandmother sat on the couch behind me with ongoing commentary on my form. Tony Little, with his long blond ponytail and form-fitting unitard, was my savior. I was jealous of the way Tony doted on Pam, his forty-year-old spandex-clad assistant. She was my nemesis, because Tony obviously had a crush on her. I could tell by the way he touched her side as he corrected her form and marveled at her youthful forty-year-old physique. One day I would be Pam, and Tony or someone like him would look at my body and admire its beauty.

I've spent the years since my second-grade revelation not eating enough, followed by periods of eating too much, all while spending hours trying to systematically deduct indulgences with exercise.

I started modeling in the third grade, and that was the first time someone who wasn't me told me I had to watch my weight.

Long before "Take Your Daughter to Work Day" existed, there was one day a year, usually the same day as the office holiday party, that the state bureaucracy factory my mother commuted four hours a day to get to and from allowed employees to bring their kids to work. Besides my birthday, it was my favorite day of the year. I was allowed to miss school; my mother bought me a new book to read on the train like a regular commuter, and once we were in her office I could spend my day making digital Christmas trees on her PC-DOS work station by strategically placing x and o characters across the page. It was about as exciting as my life got, especially since I'd had a really hard time making new friends since our move.

For the most part the commuters that took the 6:15 a.m. train to the city with my mom each morning paid me no attention—except for one woman, who periodically looked up from her magazine to smile in my direction. As we left the train she handed my mom a business card and said a few words I couldn't hear. My mother thanked her and, as we made our way to the subway, asked me if I wanted to be a model—the woman on the train was a modeling agent, she told me, and thought I was pretty. I told her that I absolutely without a doubt wanted to be a model more than anything else in the entire world.

My mother followed up with the woman, but as enthusiastic as she'd been on the train, she was no longer interested. She told my mom that her agency already had a girl who looked a lot like me and gave her the name of another agent who worked with kids—someone closer to home on Long Island. His name was Chickie, and I decided that he got that name because he really liked baby chickens. It was the only logical conclusion. My mom sent Chickie a few pictures she had taken of me on my first day of school, and shortly thereafter we were invited to come in for a formal business meet and greet.

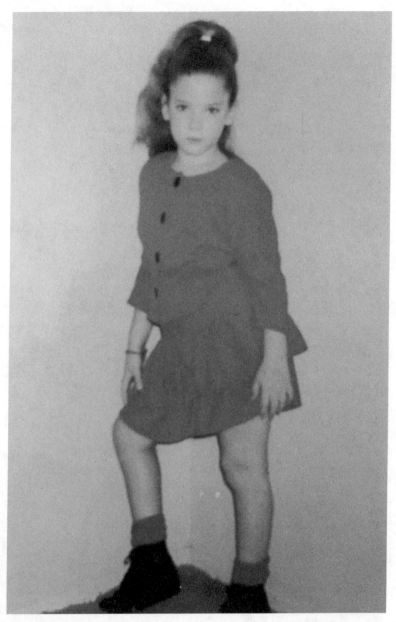

Seven years old, first day of third grade. Little did I know this picture would launch a wholly uneventful modeling career.

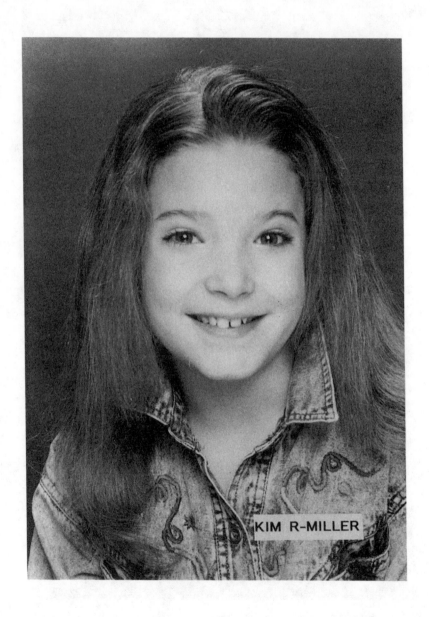

Modeling headshot.

Prior to our meeting with Chickie, I had told my only friend (and next-door neighbor) Brooke that I was going to meet with a modeling agent, and she asked if she could come along. She was two years older than I was, but she had taken me under her wing nonetheless, probably because news of my untouchable new-girl status hadn't yet reached the fifth-grade wing. We were inseparable throughout my entire third grade, and that day, we spent the rest of the afternoon pretending we were models in front of an invisible photographer.

When I went home, my mom told me emphatically that Brooke couldn't come along. I didn't understand.

"Kim, Brooke is blonde and skinny," she said. She didn't say it, but I knew that the rest the sentence was "and you're not." Noticing the disappointment on my face, she added, "If Brooke's parents want to take her to meet Chickie, I'll be happy to give them the information."

I told Brooke that she couldn't come along, making something up about only one kid being allowed in the building at a time. We never talked about my burgeoning modeling career again.

———

Chickie's office was completely unremarkable. Everything was gray: the walls, the chairs, the carpets, the desk. Even the photos of the babies and children that lined his walls came in varying shades of gray. Everything was gray except Chickie, who was wearing a burgundy suit. He didn't look like anyone I had ever seen before. He was an old man, but he didn't dress like any of the other old men that I knew. His light-pink button-down shirt had the first few buttons open, allowing his gray chest hair—what was left of it—to poke out. He wore jewelry, a lot of it, which I found shocking; I'd never seen a man wear a necklace or a ring that wasn't a wedding ring. My father didn't even wear one of those— the only ring he wore was an enormous key ring that jingled against his hip as he walked. When I was lost in a store, I could always find my dad by the sound of his keys. In my limited life experience, Chickie looked like someone from an old movie, someone who played a villain.

He didn't address my father or me at all; when we walked into his gray conference room, he gave me the once-over and proceeded to direct all his attention at my mother—she was the only one of us worth wooing.

"Nora, may I call you Nora?" he said, without giving her any real time to object. "Your daughter is lovely. She takes after you."

My dad raised an eyebrow and smirked, but he kept his eyes directed at his two thumbs—twiddling them in circles, one around the other. Being beautiful wasn't much of an accomplishment in his opinion . . . and I hadn't inherited a single physical trait from my mom. In the third grade I was already as tall as she was, and I hadn't inherited her narrow build, lean limbs, or sharp features. I looked just like my Alpine-y[4] father, blonde, broad, and pale—we looked like the kind of people who should be wearing lederhosen, not walking a runway.

"I think Kimberly could go far in this business; I could see her transitioning into TV or movies. I'd like to start sending her out right away, but she's going to need headshots."

Before we left, a premodeling to-do list established, Chickie finally spoke to me. Assessing me from across the table, he said, "You know, if you keep your weight down, you could do high fashion when you're older."

---

4.   "Alpine" was considered a sub-race of Caucasian by late nineteenth- and early twentieth-century anthropologists. It is thought that these round-faced, broadly built, short- to average-heighted, pasty-white humans migrated from Central Asia during the Neolithic revolution, and are descendants of the Celts who resided in central Europe in Neolithic times. Race was a popular topic at the turn of the twentieth century, and while still a topic of debate among some in the anthropological community, it is now widely considered a social construct (as opposed to physiological) that is lacking in evidence to explain biological variation in the species.

My clothes came from Kmart and Sears; I didn't know what "high fashion" was, but I knew enough to know that it was good and comparatively I was not. After that, I stopped eating at school and pocketed the dollar my parents gave me for lunch each day in my Mickey Mouse wallet.

While my modeling career was short-lived and fairly uneventful, my feelings about food were forever changed. It wasn't long before not eating became a game I played with myself. The less I ate, the more self-worth I was entitled to. And I wasn't unique in the slightest.

A 2015 review by Common Sense Media found that one in four children have dieted prior to the age of seven, and 80 percent of ten-year-old girls in America have already been on a diet. And these kids are creating a lifelong struggle for themselves; another study recently published in *Psychological Science* found that girls who were at a healthy medical weight but who thought of themselves as overweight were 40 percent more likely to become obese as adults than girls who had a body image that more closely reflected reality.

I certainly wasn't the first little girl to be told to watch her weight by well-meaning adults, and I wasn't the first teenaged girl to experiment with eating disorders purposefully, and I'm not the first adult to feel like I failed myself each time I regain weight I've lost. Hell, I'm probably not the last one to make a career out of losing and gaining weight ad nauseam. But why isn't this abnormal?

MISS MY HOMETOWN 1994

"Hey, K-Rae, mail!" my dad yelled from the foot of the stairs. We got a lot of mail. Actually, my mom got a lot of mail. She was responsible for all the things grown-ups were supposed to take care of in our house— things like bills and insurance and signing off on report cards—but she was also a really big fan of the TV shopping channels. She'd had spine surgery over the summer and was spending most of the year in bed healing and flipping between QVC and HSN, buying things we didn't need because there was nothing else to do, things that would inevitably end up lost in a pile of clothes, papers, and unopened boxes.

When I came home from school, I took in whatever packages UPS had left at our door and brought them upstairs, where my mother and I would open them on her bed—every afternoon a mini Christmas. My father was responsible for bringing in the mail from the mailbox. Paper was his trigger when it came to his hoarding.[1] Of course, I didn't know what hoarding was then; I just knew that he loved paper and wanted to

---

1. I talk extensively about hoarding in my family and as a mental illness in my memoir, *Coming Clean*.

give each flyer and credit card application its due inspection before my
mom could yell at him to get rid of it.

"There's something here addressed to you, kiddo," he said, handing
over the mail he didn't want to look at. I'd already gotten my issue of
Sassy magazine for the month, and it wasn't my birthday, so I couldn't
imagine who would be writing to me.

In fifth grade, the year earlier, my mother had surprised me with a
subscription to *Sassy* magazine. It was a gift for getting my first period.
I was the youngest girl in my grade but the first to "become a woman,"
which made me a minor celebrity for approximately thirty seconds. I
had inadvertently caused a scene when my period arrived exactly twelve
days after my tenth birthday.[2] Autonomy isn't big in the elementary
school code of conduct, and I knew that I'd get in trouble if I didn't ask
for my teacher's permission before going to the nurse. Up until fifth
grade I'd only had female teachers, but as luck would have it I would
have to explain my menarche to Mr. Palermo.

Mr. Palermo was a nice guy; he didn't seem to take fifth-grade melo-
drama too seriously or too personally. He'd been at it for a while, and
even though it was 1993, he still dressed like the teacher from *Welcome
Back, Kotter*, complete with demi-fro and mustache.

"Why do you need to see the nurse?" Mr. Palermo looked at me
skeptically. I was sure he thought that my combination of bathroom
and nurse was some sort of ruse to get out of the test about to take place.

"I got my prrrrrrrd," I whispered.

"Excuse me?" he said loudly.

---

2. A body-fat percentage of 17 percent is required for the onset of menarche;
    a percentage of 22 percent or higher is needed to maintain regular men-
    ses. As the average weight of American girls has increased over the last
    thirty years, it has had an inverse relationship with the onset of puberty
    and menstruation.

In a slightly louder whisper I followed up with, "When I went to the bathroom there was blood in my underwear."

The kids in the cluster of desks closest to where we were standing started laughing, and my teacher turned away from me reflexively, shooing me away with his hand, hurrying back to pretest instructions. I would have to take the spelling test during recess one day, but that would give me more time to study.

News had already spread by the time I got back to class, and for the rest of the day, I was the coolest girl in the fifth grade. It was an unexpected turn of events. I was chronically uncool and relished my new popularity. Everywhere I went, other girls asked me what it felt like. I told them it hurt. It didn't; it didn't really feel like anything at all, but I'd seen enough Midol commercials to know that pain was to be expected. Mostly I just felt like I was wearing a diaper, but I didn't want to tell them that—that was definitely something they'd make fun of me for. The nurse checked in on me throughout the day, offering me new pads and asking if I wanted to leave school early. She seemed to be just as excited about my sudden case of womanhood as my peers—I guess a first period is a lot more fun than lice checks and splinter removal. Normally I would have taken a get-out-of-school pass in a heartbeat, but I was having far too much fun being popular.

"How was school today, kiddo?" My dad was in the front yard when I got home, listening to the radio while sluggishly cleaning out the car before it was time to pick my mom up from the train station.

"Great," I said. "Guess what I got?"

"An A?" he said, already impressed.

"My period!" The euphoria of my school celebrity hadn't quite worn off.

"Huh," he said. "Okay. Call your mother." Then he went back to listening to the radio.

So far, the men in my life weren't quite as excited as I was about my newest milestone, but I knew my mom would be. I called her at work.

She cried and then, while I was still on the phone, told all her coworkers and passed on their congratulations.

"We'll go out to dinner tonight to celebrate. Decide where you want to go," she said before hanging up. She was going to try and catch an earlier train so we could start celebrating.

She'd already given me a whole speech about periods and how once I got mine, I'd be able to have a baby. I was already taller than she was and had all sorts of body hair and had been wearing a training bra for over a year. My mom had recognized the signs and had warned me it was going to happen soon, but I thought that "soon" meant in two years.

Turning ten was a big deal because I had reached double digits—I would have a double-digit age for the rest of my life. I was basically a grown-up. I had wanted to be ten for as long as I could remember, but when I'd celebrated finally reaching my inevitable goal at the bowling alley with my friends a couple of weeks earlier, I had no idea what was in store. By the end of the school year I would be wearing a C cup and would have gone through three sizes of pants to accommodate my widening hips and ever-lengthening legs.[3] I started the school year off as a kid, but by the time sixth grade started, I was five foot four inches and 120 pounds.[4] Hence, my mom's idea to subscribe me to a magazine targeted at girls going through similar things.

---

3. A 2008 study out of the Karolinska Institute in Stockholm, Sweden, found that the number of fat cells in a person's body is established during childhood and adolescence. Fat cells die at a rate of 10 percent per year, but are replaced by the same number of cells to maintain equilibrium. While a person may reduce or increase the amount of fat stored in each cell through diet and exercise, this study does much to explain why it can be especially hard for people who were overweight in childhood to lose weight as adults.

4. According to the CDC, the average height and weight of the average ten-year-old girl is 45.5 inches (four foot five inches) and around seventy pounds.

My dad handed me the letter, and I inspected it on my way upstairs to deposit the mail in my mom's room. The white envelope had a return address from Miss Junior America in bright-red cursive ink.

I tried to open the letter the way my mom did, by sliding my nail under the crease in the paper and slipping it along the seam. It always looked so graceful when she did it. I usually ended up tearing the paper and giving myself a paper cut, and this time was no exception.

I sucked on my bloody index finger as I read the letter from Miss Junior America. She had written to tell me that some anonymous admirer of my beauty had recommended me to represent my hometown in the New York State Pre-Teen Pageant. It didn't actually say what my hometown was, it just said "your hometown," which I thought was strange. Obviously Miss Junior America knew what my hometown was; it was on the envelope. No matter, there was someone out there who wanted me to be a beauty queen. A beauty queen like Kelly Kapowski.

Tiffani Amber Thiessen's face was printed right in the middle of the letter, with a tiny italicized blurb explaining that she had won the national pageant five years earlier, right before she started filming *Saved by the Bell*. Kelly Kapowski / Tiffani Amber Thiessen was the ultimate. There was no one in the world I could want to be more than Kelly Kapowski; she made sweatshirts look cool. Thanks to my very own beauty pageant Magwitch, this could be my big break too. The New York State pageant would be judged by two casting directors and an acting agent. I was going to be famous.

I just had to convince my mother.

I was never very good at playing it cool, so I barreled into her room with the mail and launched onto her bed to hand her the letter.

"Can I pleeeeeeze?"

"Can you please, what?" She took the letter and started reading, her face slowly turning from relaxed to mildly angry.

"Do you know who recommended you?" she asked.

"No." I was just as curious as she was. I hoped it was my acting teacher or one of my dance teachers.

"Do you think it was your pervert teacher?" she asked. My sixth grade math and science teacher told me in front of the class that my barely audible voice was "very sexy" but that I needed to speak louder. I promptly stopped speaking altogether.

"No, he got fired for slapping Colin," I said. Actually, he hadn't been fired so much as it had been strongly recommended by the school board that he retire at the end of the school year. I didn't think he was much of a pageant nominator.

"You're not doing this," she said.

"What's the difference between this and modeling?"

In my nine-month tenure as a child model, I had booked only one job, a commercial for a household cleaner, but when I got to the house the producers had rented for the shoot, I found out I'd been replaced by a dog. I still got paid for the day, and I got to eat all the craft services I wanted, so it wasn't a total loss. After a while I got sick of being pulled out of school for auditions; the kids in my class didn't believe that I was a model and made fun of me for saying I was, so I gave up my fledgling career in product placement and returned to life as a normal eight-year-old.

"The money you made modeling[5] went away for college. This pageant costs more than our last car."

In the ten minutes that I had known that I was beauty-queen material, I realized that I wanted to be Miss "My Hometown" more than I had ever wanted anything else before. This letter wasn't just going to change my life; it was going to change all our lives. Once I was a famous actress I'd be able to buy my parents a new house; we'd have a maid

---

5.   I did actually make a couple grand for sitting around the commercial shoot not being a dog, money that eventually paid for my college textbooks.

to clean up after Dad and an in-ground pool for my mom to do her physical therapy in. I just needed to convince my mother that this was an investment in our future.

The next week of our lives was an all-out assault. Since my mother was still recovering from the surgeries that had cut through her abdominal and back muscles, she didn't have the strength to get out of bed without help, which meant she was a captive audience to all my whining, pleading, promising, badgering, and guilt. My father didn't care one way or another; as long as I continued being alive and left him alone to listen to NPR, he supported my doing whatever I wanted. My mom was the decision maker in our family. And I knew I could wear her down. She showed a crack in her armor at one point, mentioning feeling guilty for being in bed for the majority of my sixth-grade year, and I used it to my advantage, promising her that when she was stronger in the summer, we would be able to spend time together practicing and preparing. This wouldn't just be my beauty pageant; this would be our summer of mother-daughter bonding. Eventually she ceded, either out of understanding, exhaustion, annoyance, or guilt. I didn't care why: I was going to the pageant.

As far as bonding activities go, spending the summer preparing for a beauty pageant was financially akin to going to a ritzy sleepaway camp—the kind of camp we couldn't afford. There was an entry fee, tickets to a fancy mandatory dinner, and a reservation at a much nicer hotel than we'd ever stayed at before. We also had to prepay for a photography package and buy an evening gown. The pageant packet that Miss Junior America sent to me after I sent them my entry fee strongly suggested we hire one of their professional makeup artists, but my mother informed me that that would be happening over her dead body, as would the optional swimsuit competition.

With each check she wrote, my mother promised to find whoever it was that recommended me for the pageant and give them a piece of her mind and a bill of our expenses.

The pageant was at the beginning of August, and school wrapped up at the end of June. My mom and I had a little over a month to get everything ready. After my last day of school, my father drove us to a discount bridal salon near my dance studio to pick out a dress. I wanted to try on a wedding dress, just for fun, but the woman who worked there told me that I would need an engagement ring first, so I headed over to the section where they kept the colorful kids' gowns. Since I was built like a twenty-five-year-old, the hot-pink sequin-adorned tulle dresses that they normally reserved for pageant girls didn't fit me. I needed an adult gown, so I was quickly redirected to the bridesmaid section. Long green dresses with fabric flowers, burgundy off-the-shoulder cocktail attire, and black velvet strapless numbers filled the rack.

"Do you have anything a little more age appropriate?" my mom asked the sales clerk.

"Hmmm, I may have something in the back. Hold on." And she was gone. I thought I might go check out the wedding dresses in her absence, but my mom held my hand firmly in place, since I had a habit of breaking things that she later had to purchase.

The woman came out holding a plantation-style dress in peach satin and white lace that looked like it came right out of a nineties retelling of *Gone with the Wind*.

"Someone put a deposit on this and changed their mind," she said.

I couldn't imagine why anyone would abandon such a beautiful creation. It was perfect, right down to the iridescent sequins sewn into the bodice. It cost $350, but I didn't want to look at any other dresses. I knew it was a lot of money; I was still under the impression that owning $100 meant that you were rich, so I couldn't imagine that we could ever afford such a luxurious item, but I was in love.

"Go ahead; try it on," my mom said. And I ran for the dressing rooms.

It was a little loose, but a pretty close fit.

"Alterations are included," the saleswoman chirped as my mother and I stared at one another in the mirror. I didn't want to say I wanted it, because it was so expensive, but I wanted it, and I willed my mother to read my mind.

"You look beautiful," she said with a resolved smile. "You're going to get married in this dress."

"I will. I will. I will," I lied. No one gets married in peach satin; everyone knows that.

I hugged my mom and skipped out to the car to tell my dad that we'd just spent more on one dress than his entire wardrobe was worth. He just shook his head, raised an eyebrow, and went back to listening to NPR.

———

I would not be participating in the talent competition because that cost extra, and the bathing suit competition was off the table because my mom said so. Since I was opting out of two of the five segments of the competition, I knew that I needed to shine in the interview, sporting wear, and evening gown sections.

My parents mock-interviewed me about my interests during car rides, and at night I would recite my evening-wear speech to myself alone in my room while I practiced smiling confidently yet demurely at myself in the mirror, like the women I'd seen in the Miss America pageant. The only thing I didn't have was a Miss Pre-Teen Anywhere–appropriate body.

I didn't like having breasts or getting attention from men who were old enough to know better, and my wardrobe consisted mostly of baggy carpenter jeans and oversized T-shirts and sweaters. I knew my everyday attire wouldn't impress the judges: Miss Junior America was glamorous and ladylike; she didn't shop in the men's section of Old Navy. I loved feminine, form-fitting clothes; I just didn't like wearing them in public. Whenever I wore something trendy to school, I felt like an imposter. I wasn't small and delicate like the popular girls. I was broad and curva-ceous and looked like an adult. I was going to stand out on stage against all of those age-appropriately sized preteens from around the state.

My mom called the pageant to ask if I could switch to the teen competition, assuring them that even though I was entering seventh grade, I would fit in better with the high schoolers. They said no, that it wouldn't be fair to me to be judged against more mature girls.

My prepageant high was replaced by a crisis of confidence. I wanted to be Miss Pre-Teen Junior America; I just wanted to be her in some-one else's body, and I spent a week crying and begging my mom to do something, anything to make it better.

"I will let you go on a diet for one week," my mom said while we ate dinner at the edge of her bed. I had already sniveled my way through an entire *Lois & Clark* rerun.

"But I am on a diet," I told her. I was always on a diet of my own making, and at this particular moment in my diet narrative I believed that I could eat anything I wanted as long as it was fat-free.

"There's a diet I did when I was younger; it's called the Stillman Diet," she told me. "I'll let you do it, but not for more than a week. It's not healthy."

———

Dr. Irwin Maxwell Stillman was a small, thin man who bore a striking resemblance to the old Perdue Chicken guy. He looked like someone's grandfather: caring, trustworthy, a family doctor in Coney Island for forty-five years. America fell in love with him in 1967 when his revo-lutionary plan for rapid weight loss was published. It was called *The Doctor's Quick Weight Loss Diet* but everyone called it the Stillman Diet in honor of its namesake, and it promised "permanent, joyful weight loss."

Stillman claimed to have treated over ten thousand overweight patients in his forty-five years as a general practitioner with his "foolproof" diet, making him quite possibly the most popular physician in the history of family medicine. Although not an original concept—that would be credited to Dr. Max Rubner and later to Dr. Eugene DuBois—Stillman's plan was based on Dr. DuBois's (the same doctor who presided over Vilhjalmur Stefansson's Inuit-diet experiment) theory of specific dynamic action. DuBois claimed that the body required up to 30 percent more energy to digest protein than it did carbohydrates and fat, making the simple act of digesting protein a metabolism-boosting form of exercise.

Stillman's plan was simple, if not excruciatingly boring, requiring followers to eat a low-fat diet consisting of nothing but very lean meats, fat-free cottage cheese, eggs, and eight glasses of water a day. He boasted that if they followed the plan correctly, a dieter would lose up to fifteen pounds in their first week, and a pound a day after.

While Stillman is often cited as the father of the high-protein era, he was actually about one hundred years too late to claim that title. William Banting, a well-to-do British coffin maker, was the world's first diet-book author and high(ish)-protein-diet advocate. While a man of five foot five inches and 202 pounds wouldn't seem at all shocking today, in 1862 Banting was a spectacle of obesity. He wrote, "I could not stoop to tie my shoes, so [to] speak, nor to attend to the little offices humanity requires without considerable pain and difficulty which only the corpulent can understand; I have been compelled to go downstairs slowly backward to save the jar of increased weight on the knee and ankle joints, and have been obliged to puff and blow over every slight exertion, particularly that of going upstairs."

It was while being treated for hearing loss that Banting first met Dr. William Harvey, a renowned aural surgeon, who seemed to be more fascinated by Banting's size than ears. Harvey had only recently returned to London from a Paris lecture about the treatment of diabetes with diet. The study of diabetes was still in its infancy, and the concept of a sugarlike secretion emitted from the liver was only a theory, but the ideas discussed by French physiologist Claude Bernard fascinated him. Banting was desperate for help, and Harvey was curious about the effects of fat, sugar, and starches on the body. The two were perfect for one another.

At Harvey's suggestion, Banting ate only small portions of lean meat, fruits and vegetables, a small amount of dry toast, and a hefty amount of wine and/or gin. Within a year Banting had lost forty-eight pounds and was a trim 154 pounds. While a weight loss of less than a pound a week would have had Banting booted from *The Biggest Loser* house in no time, it was a substantial weight loss that was revolutionary for its time. So enthralled with his new svelte physique and low-carb lifestyle was he that in 1863 he used his considerable fortune to fund a self-published booklet, *Letter on Corpulence Addressed to the Public*, which he gave out free of charge to anyone who was interested. At first.

Banting's letter became so popular that he would eventually need to start charging for it, printing what would become the world's first diet book. Word of this high-protein diet spread around the world, and for the next fifty years, dieting would be referred to socially as "Banting."

Banting was old news by 1994. To be honest, so was Stillman, but since I was too young at eleven to drink the six glasses of spirits a day that Banting's diet required, Stillman was my man. I didn't care if it was safe; I would do anything. Surely the fact that I was young would be a buffer from any less-than-stellar aftereffects. My mother went on the diet with me for moral support but was skeptical I'd be able to stick to something so restrictive. She was wrong: I loved the rigidity and lack of choice that Stillman stipulated. It may not have been my first diet, but it was my first taste of real deprivation. It was awful but amazing. By the second day of eating only protein, I lost my appetite. By the fifth day I could taste the stomach acid in my mouth as I choked down the turkey burger, without catsup, my mother had brought to a friend's birthday

BBQ for me—explaining that I wouldn't be eating the hamburgers and hot dogs the rest of the kids were having. By the very last day, I hardly left my bed. Not because I felt sick, but because I loved the way my rib cage poked out when I was lying flat on my back. I spent all day running my hands up and down the hollow between my ribs and belly. I felt empty. Hunger had always made me feel uncomfortable before but now I loved it. That feeling of emptiness meant I had succeeded. By the time we left for the hotel in Rye Brook, I had lost eight pounds. Less than I wanted, less than my mom promised I would. I still looked like a woman, but I was far less concerned about my breasts and hips as I was completely enamored with the smallness of my waist.

As soon as we checked into the hotel, I ran to the full-length mirror (of which we didn't have any at home) in our room, lifted up my shirt, and proceeded to watch my stomach all but completely disappear from the side as I held in my stomach, then watched it reappear each time I took a breath. Ribs, I loved the way my ribs stuck out. I could count them. I wanted to look like that all the time.

We met a girl from the teen pageant in the hallway; her name was Patricia, and many years later I would see her representing the state of Pennsylvania in either the Miss America or Miss USA pageant.[6] My

---

6. When the Miss America pageant started in the 1920s, the average contestant had a healthy BMI between twenty and twenty-five. The average waist size of a contestant in 1921 was twenty-six inches, with the winner clocking in at a short five foot one inch. Now Miss America contestants have twenty-four-inch waists and heights ranging from five foot six inches to five foot eleven inches. In the last ninety-five years, contestants' body weight has decreased by 12 percent. According to a report in *The Journal of the American Medical Association*, an increasing number of recent winners had BMIs under 18.5, the border between normal and underweight. In 2014, Indiana's Miss USA contestant, Mekayla Diehl, was lauded by the media for having a more "realistic" figure: the beauty queen was five foot eight inches and a size four with a BMI of eighteen, which is considered technically underweight.

mother told her we'd never done this before, and she took me under her wing. She came to our room before the show to help me get dressed and give me tips on impressing the judges. And even though she was prepping for her own pageant, she ducked into the ballroom with the stage to watch me give my evening-gown speech. Patricia was graduating from high school at the end of the next school year, and I was completely enamored by her. She was everything I wanted to be: a teenager, beautiful in an easy, all-American kind of way, kind, friendly. She didn't seem to overthink everything—she just did the right thing and looked perfect doing it. I wasn't like that at all. I overthought everything. I thought things out so much that I would miss my chance to do anything at all, and everything I did have the gumption to do was labored and self-conscious. I made up my mind that I would pretend to be Patricia while I was on stage. I knew I wouldn't win, but I would pretend that I belonged there.

Any delusions I had of winning were shattered when I saw the girls I was competing against, with their tailor-made costumes and professional makeup artists. I had a wrinkled skort, a plantation dress, and the little bit of lip gloss my mom let me wear. They gave speeches about being good in school; I gave a speech about creating systematic help for sexually abused children in the public school system. Everything about me was wrong for the pageanting world, but I was more confident than I'd ever been before. I felt thin, and that was the most important thing. I'd never felt more beautiful than I had standing in front of that full-length mirror, my shirt pulled up, looking at my ribs.

THE KING AND I
(GO TO FAT CAMP)

No one knows for sure what William the Conqueror looked like, but rumor has it he was fat. The majority of the paintings depicting his grandeur, and more importantly stature, were commissioned a half century or more after his death, and they vary between depicting a lithe moonfaced warrior king and a Henry VIII doppelgänger sporting a toga. What we do know from a lone femur saved of the king's remains was that he was about five foot ten inches—pretty darn tall for the eleventh century. In his treatise of William I's life, *William the Conqueror: The Norman Impact upon England*, late historian of the Norman era David C. Douglas recounts the lore that when William's tomb was opened for the first time in 1522, what remained was the well-preserved, albeit appropriately decayed, carrion of what appeared to be "a large man with notably long arms and legs."

I don't have remarkably long legs or arms, but other than that, the king and I have a lot in common, and I've taken him on as something of a totemic ancestor.[1] We were both born out of wedlock, we both descended from Vikings (I actually have no proof on my part, but I sure look it), we're both bad at riding horses, and we both went to fat camp. I have a soft spot for one of the most brutal rulers in England's history. Sure, he liked to cut off the hands and feet of people who mocked his less-than-kosher birthright, and he starved more than a hundred thousand of his own countrymen to show his dominance and earn their fealty, but deep down I know he was just a wounded soul.

While lore has it that William ate scarcely, and it has been suggested that his lifelong struggle with his weight may have been the result of a metabolic disorder, I wouldn't blame him if he did indulge in some emotional eating. His father, Robert the Magnificent (or Robert the Devil, depending on whom you ask or which history books you read), died shortly after inheriting the dukedom, leaving eight-year-old William the leader of Normandy. This job title led to immediate and incessant attempts on the young duke's life—his childhood caretakers were murdered, one after the other, including one poor soul who was sleeping in bed with the future king when he had his throat slit, and kid-William woke up next to a bloody dead body. William managed to survive his childhood and went on to conquer different French provinces and eventually all of England.[2] But despite his accomplishments, he was considered a generally unpleasant fellow, and his weight was oft the butt of courtly jokes. He was particularly picked on by the king of France, Philip the Amorous (best royal nickname), who referred to William as "lying in," as in a very pregnant woman who can't move about comfortably.

---

1.   I'm most likely not related to William I, but you might be. Steve Jones, Welsh geneticist, author, and professor of genetics at the Galton Laboratory at University College London, suggests an estimated 25 percent of the British population are members of William's gene pool in his book *In the Blood: God, Genes and Destiny* (HarperCollins, 1996).
2.   There's a lot more to it, but this isn't his memoir.

According to some accounts, the corpulent conqueror became despondent when he got too big to fit in his bathtub or ride a horse without "breaking it in half" and devised a weight-loss plan that consisted of lying in bed and eating nothing at all; his only sustenance came in the form of alcohol—the first weight-loss diet in recorded history.[3] Remarkably, he did lose some weight, since he eventually was able to return to horseback riding—which he did so he could go to fat camp.

It was in 1087, and William the Bastard, as he was often referred to, was en route to a spa in Rouen, France,[4] for a weight-loss regimen when his horse bucked so abruptly and assiduously that the king was thrust into the pommel of his saddle, rupturing his intestines. After his accident the king was taken to the priory of Saint Gervase in Rouen, where he lay dying of his infected wounds. He was accompanied by his closest confidants and two sons, Henry and William, until he had offered them their inheritance, at which point his chamber was ransacked and the king was left to die alone.

King William's alcohol-only diet[5] didn't seem to have changed his girth that much, as evidenced by the fact that the king did not fit in his coffin. As the church attendants tasked with preparing his body for burial smashed and smooshed his unembalmed, bacteria-riddled belly into his coffin, it became evident that William was too rotund to close the casket, and so he had an unplanned open-casket funeral.

---

3. Alcohol is actually terrible for weight loss: it has seven calories per gram, almost twice as much as protein or carbohydrates, which have four, and only moderately less than fat, which has nine.

4. William was probably much more comfortable in France, as he never actually learned to speak English, despite being king. His primary tongue was French.

5. Alcohol-based diets came back in vogue in the three-martini-lunch era of the 1960s. In 1964, Robert Cameron published *The Drinking Man's Diet*, which promoted low-carb eating with the exception of alcohol.

It was a hot July day, and the heat, combined with the pressure caused by his tight quarters and the fermenting bacteria in his body, built throughout the ceremony until he exploded, releasing pus and a stench that forced the mourners to flee and the bishops presiding over the funeral service to do a quick prayer and follow suit. And so came to an ignominious end the first Norman king of England.

If William the Conqueror's story isn't a cautionary tale against extreme, gimmick-based diets, I don't know what is. But as far as weight loss goes, William was the first "celebrity" to diet openly, and despite the existence of medieval French weight-loss clinics, the subject of dieting would not be discussed in public record again for quite a few centuries.

In his book *Never Satisfied: A Cultural History of Diets, Fantasies and Fat*, Hillel Schwartz notes that the archetypal public dieters were more often male until late in the nineteenth century. Dieting, he found, was considered a "masculine" act of willfulness until the onset of the Victorian era, when it became a female art form.

Like the first Norman king of England, I too believed that running away to a weight-loss retreat would solve all my problems. After *Sassy's* demise, my puberty-centric magazine subscription was changed to *YM* (*Young and Modern*). It was a generally fluffier read than *Sassy* had been, but I read each issue devoutly. My favorite sections were the horoscopes (being a Capricorn, my horoscope was chronically schoolwork related, but I remained hopeful something exciting might happen) and the ads. The pages that littered the back of each and every issue of *YM* were throwaways: hokey photos of friendship bracelets, hair crimpers, plastic jewelry, and matching American Girl doll / actual, real-life girl pajama sets. They were pages that served no other purpose than to dispose of used gum in, but in my early teen years they were just as important as the articles about why I needed espadrilles, how to minimize a break-out in minutes, and surefire ways to get my crush to like me (which

I had no interest in because that would require me to actually talk to him). Interspersed between the various tchotchkes for sale were ads for weight-loss camps across the country.

I was obsessed with fat camp. I could spend hours inspecting the various flavors the camps came in. Some promised the college experience: spending the summer in a university's dorms, using the fitness center, and eating in the cafeteria. Others promised a woodsy affair, offering a traditional sleepaway camp with nature-based activities. Some boasted hotel accommodations and daily maid service. All of them promised I would make friendships that would last a lifetime and, more importantly, return to my real life a more beautiful and confident me than I'd ever been before.

It was a montage in the making: I could go off to spend the summer laughing with new friends over lush salads and will-testing, sweat-drenching step aerobics, and when I came back to school in the fall it would be with a totally new persona. Not only would I be a lean, willowy Kim, but one with an impeccable sense of fashion who was also outgoing and socially skillful. I would be someone else entirely.

When the dog-eared yellowing magazine pages no longer satisfied, I called and asked for brochures from every camp that advertised my gateway to eternal happiness. It took a few months to work up the nerve to call, because I knew that once someone answered on the other line, I would have admitted that I was fat, that I had failed at being beautiful. The ladies and answering machines on the other end never seemed to care much about my emotional journey; they took down my name and address, and a short while later I was flush in fat-camp brochures. I kept them in a neat pile by my bed, stealing moments between homework assignments and TV shows to go on little fantasy excursions.

Fat camp wasn't going to happen, though. Kids from my town didn't go away to camp; if they went to camp at all, it was to the YMCA while their parents were at work.

I asked once, over dinner, sitting at the foot of my mother's bed while the TV played in the background. Since my indoctrination to fad diets before the pageant, I'd become obsessed with diets. I knew how easy it was to lose weight, and I wanted to do it all the time. I just also wanted to eat food sometimes too, which is why I always gained it back.

"What if I went away for the summer?" I said, during the commercial break.

"Where are you going?" my mom asked.

"Camp. I've never been to camp. There are a few camps upstate where you can lose weight," I told my parents. "You take exercise classes during the day, and you have no choice but to stick to the diet because diet food is all they give you."

"I don't think you need fat camp, kiddo," my dad chimed in. He was always really unsupportive.

My mom was more utilitarian. "Sleepaway camp is for people who don't like their kids. I like you. You're staying here."

And that was it. My mother's answer was immutable. I was doomed to a life of self-prescribed diets and a half hour of ab-rolling to La Bouche's "Be My Lover" on repeat before bed each night.

Summers transitioned from bike riding and ice-cream trucks to wine coolers and waitressing shifts, and I eventually forgot about my dreams of spending a summer transforming into my ideal self.

Near the end of my senior year, after finals but before the actual end of school, when all that was left to do was watch movies and wait to graduate, I took the day off to visit my aunt Lee. Since my aunt had never had kids of her own, nor wanted them, I pretty much served as the communal family offspring. Aunt Lee lived in Manhattan, and visiting her was like a day with the ghost of my future grown-up life; the city was infinitely more my speed than the suburbs. It was loud and busy, and I felt safe in how easily I could get lost among the crowds. Aunt Lee took me to shows and to eat at trendy restaurants, and in between, we'd walk around neighborhoods that were intimidatingly cool, neighborhoods I planned on living in one day.

"If you're interested," she told me, "I'd like to send you to Camp Charlemagne[6] as a graduation present." She must have remembered my obsession with fat camp—it was middle-school me's dream come true. But it wasn't the no-brainer it would have been five years earlier. It was the summer between high school and college. I wanted to spend the summer with my friends, and I needed to work. College was expensive and I was paying for it on my own. But it was a generous offer, and I desperately wanted to start college off thin. Reruns of my middle-school fantasies of leaving at the beginning of the summer an ugly duckling and returning to my real life a beautiful swan started to play in my mind while Aunt Lee told me about the camp.

Thin trumped everything else. It always had. So even though I would miss my friends and would have to take out extra loans for school, I knew I couldn't say no—this was a once-in-a-lifetime opportunity.

My parents refused to drive me to camp—I'd gone against their wishes and was relegated to taking the bus to some town in upstate New York with lots of trees and a surprising lack of strip malls. Fat-camp bus started in New York City, then hit all the major area airports: LaGuardia and JFK in Queens, Newark in New Jersey. Kids were flying in from all over for their fresh start, and as the bus filled up with children far younger than I was, I knew I'd made a terrible mistake. I was too old to be a sleepaway-camp newbie. I hadn't even left the metro area and I was already feeling homesick, which only amplified when I got to my cabin. My cabin was full of chipper girls who'd been coming to this camp since before puberty, and all knew one another. These were girls who came

6. Names have been changed to protect the author from any possibility of being added to a fat-camp alumni page.

from families who had no problem dropping a few grand so their kids would be forced to count calories. And all five of my roommates were much bigger than I was, which made me question the effectiveness of the camp—I was at least thirty pounds lighter than my smallest bunk-mate, and I wasn't exactly a waif. None of them seemed bothered by the fact that there were six of us in one room and that our shower was a wall-mounted garden hose in a mildew-covered plywood hut. This was camping. This is what I'd always wanted.

The first order of fat-camp business was to change into our bath-ing suits and head to the main hall, not for swimming but for "before" pictures and a weigh-in. There were hundreds of us, shy, self-conscious kids, some who looked far too young to be on a diet—not that I was one to judge—waiting in line for our chance to pose for the most awk-ward school photos ever. I felt like I had some sort of responsibility as an almost adult to the younger campers, the ones who looked like I felt, like they just wanted to go home, to pretend I was comfortable standing around in my Speedo.

I had never been in a mess hall, but figured it couldn't be that differ-ent from a school cafeteria. If only. I didn't know how much my aunt paid for this all-inclusive experience, but I knew it was a lot. So when I entered the mess hall, I expected there to be slightly more refined fare than your average cafeteria. I wasn't a snob: my food choices at home weren't all that great—we hadn't used our kitchen for years, and the downstairs of our house had all but been abandoned to the garbage that had taken over our home thanks to my father's hoarding. But as I stood in line for pita bread with Spam Lite and vegetable lasagna that was mostly cheese, I realized that . . . health food it wasn't. What hap-pened to all the gourmet food I had read about all those years earlier in beautifully illustrated pamphlets? Where was the perfectly grilled chicken breast with steamed asparagus and brightly colored tropical fruit salad? It was all a lie, and I refused to eat dinner. I would not eat canned-ham tacos. I didn't hate myself that much.

When I woke up the next morning, I realized that I was still there. And I would be for the next two weeks, so it was time to make the most of it. The first call of order was facing the fact that fat camp wasn't what I wanted it to be, so I'd have to be proactive. I knew my way around a diet, and the powdered eggs, pancakes, and grape Kool-Aid-esque concoction that made up breakfast wasn't going to help me start my college life in prime form. I skipped breakfast. I wasn't there for the food.

The rest of the day was a grab bag of aerobics-based electives, a nutrition class, and a group game. I started every morning with a group Tae Bo video, about a hundred of us packed into a gym, doing our best not to punch one another while we flailed about trying to mimic the enormous Billy Blanks projected on the wall. When Tae Bo was over, I walked over to the step aerobics, which took place in a carport under the trees. Our instructor couldn't have been much older than I was, and she seemed just as uncomfortable shouting out instructions to a bunch of out-of-breath teenagers as I did jumping around in a forest full of strangers. There was no escaping the awkwardness that was a bunch of overweight kids doing aerobics outside in the middle of July.

I was supposed to make lifelong friends, but I wasn't gregarious by nature, nor was I sure I really wanted to be friends with my fellow campers.

Immediately upon arrival I was given the nickname Lil Kim. Usually a nickname is a good sign when it comes to social acceptance. In this case it wasn't symbolic of my having ingratiated myself to the natives or that I reminded them of the pint-sized rapper or even an assessment of my overall size. I was called Lil Kim because of my spatial relation to the other Kim. She was new too, and she never stood a chance. Once introductions were made and bunk assignments sorted, it was clear that Big Kim was screwed. Big Kim was close to six foot two inches and in her mid to late twenties, too old to belong. Like me, she was socially awkward and had come to camp hoping to turn a corner in her life. Being thin would make everything better—that's why we were all there. But unlike me she couldn't just keep her head down until camp was over. She was too tall, too outside the norm for the gang of girls who had already claimed the camp as their own.

I found one friend, another newcomer to Camp Charlemagne. Robin was the only girl in the "adult" camper group who was smaller than I was. By all accounts, she was skinny. According to her, her parents sent her to a new camp every year so they could travel without worrying that she was getting into trouble. They didn't put much thought into it, so they just picked a place and sent a check—Camp Charlemagne was the only camp they could find to send their legally adult daughter, which was how a ninety-pound college sophomore had ended up at fat camp. My mom may have been onto something with her earlier judgment of sleepaway camp: some people just didn't like their kids.

Robin and I paired up for power walks and group Red Rover games, but went our separate ways when it came time to do cardio. I needed a real calorie burn; she preferred not to sweat. We had nothing in common: she talked about her boyfriend incessantly, and I wanted to calculate our caloric expenditures. We probably wouldn't have connected outside of camp, but we'd seen what happened to Big Kim and knew that we each needed an ally.

The seasoned campers had formed their cliques years earlier; they had history, inside jokes, and favorite activities that they congregated around. They didn't seem to mind my existence, and I did my best not to invade their space, which was good because they could be vicious. Maybe they were just lashing back at the world. Maybe they were always mean. Whatever it was, I wasn't there to make friends. I just wanted to go to step class.

***

By the time my two-week fat-camp adventure was over, I was actually psyched to hit the scale. I'd spent a cumulative fifty-six hours exercising and had survived on ice pops and salad, the only mess-hall items I could stomach. I was sure that I was at least ten pounds lighter, and so on my last day of camp I met with the nutrition staff to review my "life plan" and find out what my effort had earned me.

I was up an eighth of a pound.

"Oh, don't worry, honey," the counselor told me. "It's all muscle."

TWO

BUTTS AND BELLIES

Another date with the lovely but chunky Kimberly. I'm trying to decide if I'm being infantile and superficial, since so far she's pretty much perfect in every way that counts, or is it a legitimate deal breaker? Aside from being smart and sharp and witty and successful, she's genuinely beautiful and is great in bed. But she does have a big butt and a belly, which do bother me. On one hand there's always going to be something about the other person, and I'd rather it be a perfect mental match than physical, and altogether I am attracted to her. I've

> dated a lot of women the past few years
> and so far she really does stand out. On
> the other hand, she has a big butt and a
> belly, which bother me, and as you said,
> it's likely to only get worse. So I'm not
> sure what I want to do . . .

The good news is that I'm good in bed. I've always wondered about that.

The bad news is that I fell in love with someone who wasn't sure whether my problem areas were his deal breakers.

I don't know why I started reading Roy's email.

Actually, I do know why I started reading his email. I didn't trust him, since it was by email that I had found out that Paul had cheated on me. Paul and I had been together for almost four years. He was the first man I slept with, my first boyfriend, the first man I loved—in that order. At twenty-one I just wanted to lose my virginity before it became an embarrassing accessory; love I was a little more reticent about.

I hadn't actually dated before Paul—it hadn't even occurred to me that I might want to have a romantic relationship until after I'd graduated from college. I didn't have enough scars to be jaded, and I didn't have enough sense after four years together to not trust him when he started spending weeks at a time in the DC suburb he hailed from, visiting his family. Even when all his phone conversations inevitably came back to Danielle, the new paralegal at his father's firm, I just assumed he loved his family and was glad to spend some time with a young person while helping out at the family business.

I trusted him completely.

After he returned from another two-week stint in DC, she sent me an email, to my work email address, titled "I thought you should know." It included a series of steamy IM chats and emails in which they discussed their sex life, her long legs, and the things they wanted to do to one another.

Why would she send this to me at work?

My first reaction is always rational, practical. A calm before my emotional storm. I just wanted to be at home instead of in a cubicle while reading about their penchant for obscure bands as mood music, compliments on feats of sexual expertise, or apologies about embarrassing mishaps. But that didn't stop me from reading. They talked about going to Cuba together, about mashed-potato massages (an inside joke, I assumed, not a sensual aid), about me—about how I'd come to surprise him one weekend and ruined their plans. It sunk in; my boyfriend was sleeping with someone else. A lot, it seemed, based on what I was reading. I forwarded him the email, explaining that my work email—probably the only one she could find on the Internet—was an inappropriate venue for this sort of revelation, before I started crying at my desk. *I'm going home now,* I wrote as my final salutation. And then I told my boss, tears and snot streaming down my face, that I needed to go home for the day—I wasn't feeling well.

Paul's reply was almost instantaneous. My BlackBerry started flashing before I'd even made it to the elevator bank. I stood frozen, phone in hand, in the building lobby as I took each sentence in, digesting and repeating and torturing myself with it before moving on to the next.

I've fucked up.

You fucked her.

Here's the thing. This, whatever it was, is over. It was very short-lived, and it's done. I was depressed about life and about us. I thought I wanted out, so I set about to sabotage things.

I thought of reasons he'd be depressed about in life, about us, but in the four years we'd been together we'd never even had a fight. Our life, our relationship, was so completely status quo. We read the *New York Times* together in bed on Sunday mornings, talked politics at local bars, sang karaoke in Koreatown, and went on vacation with couple friends. We spent holidays with his family and talked about our future, about hypothetical kids and the hypothetical apartments we'd live in— together—one day. You don't cheat on people you're planning a future with.

> But what I learned was that I don't want to sabotage things. I only want you. I love you more now than ever. I'm sorry.

> All I can do now is put my fate in your hands.

On the subway home I reread their emails over and over, arming myself with the details of their relationship.

I wondered how many times. How many times had I called him and wished him sweet dreams via voice mail while he was having sex with her? I was so stupid. So stupid.

By the time I came home Paul was already there, pacing in front of my building's gate. We lived two blocks from one another. I'd wanted to move in together after we'd been dating for three years. Paul said he wasn't ready.

I was sure my landlord was going to yell at him—she yelled at everyone from her lawn chair on the balcony, a throwback to old-school Brooklyn, complete with muumuu. She didn't yell, but she did stare at him from her perch, shaking her head in disapproval.

As Paul walked the same four feet over and over, he ran his hands through his dark hair, repeatedly, hysterically. I watched him from the corner of my block for a few seconds, deciding if I could handle the coming confrontation. He looked delinquent. He wanted me to see how tormented he was. He'd always had a flair for the dramatic. When he saw me coming toward him, he extended his arms to me, offering me a pint of coffee-flavored Häagen-Dazs, my favorite. It was still solid; he hadn't been there long.

I took the ice cream and let him in. I didn't say anything; it wasn't my responsibility to talk. I just sat down on my couch and watched while he curled up into a tight ball on my living room floor and cried. He promised me that it was over between them and asked me if I would hit him. If I hit him he would feel better, he told me. I shook my head no. I didn't want to hit him, and I didn't want him to feel better. I just watched his performance as he bewailed needing to be with her to prove to himself that he really wanted to be with me.

"Why her?"

These were the only words I could manage to say. What did she have that I didn't have? I knew I sounded like a cliché, but I didn't understand. I had always been such a people pleaser, such a Paul pleaser. I spent four years trying to make him happy. I just needed to know where I failed.

"I don't know," he told me. "I liked her body. She's small. Thin."

A week after we broke up he dropped off a box of my things that I'd left at his apartment: deodorant, toothbrush, hairbrush, pajamas—four years, four items. And he left a note along with a box of chocolates: "I hope your future is sweet." The chocolates had already been pilfered, all the good ones missing. My apology was a half-eaten box of chocolates and a pint of coffee ice cream.

When I went back to work the next day, my boss called me into her office. She gave me a box of tissues to keep on my desk, asked if I was okay, and then said, "When you're ready I'd like to introduce you to my son." She hadn't believed that I was sick.

I never met my boss's son. I took some time off dating, and when I did venture back into the world of getting-to-know-yous, it never

amounted to anything serious; I never let it. My life was too complicated, and no matter how much I liked someone, no matter how good
they looked on paper or what promises they made me, trust was off
the table.

In the three years after Paul and I broke up, I'd dated a lot of really
great guys and a few not-so-great guys. Each time I reminded myself
that they weren't him. They had never knowingly hurt me, but that
didn't seem to matter to the part of my brain that allowed me to feel
comfortable letting my guard down around men who might want to
see me naked one day.

Danielle was small. She was thin and I was not. There were millions
of Danielles out there, and as much as the Pauls of the world loved curling up at night with my personality, I couldn't give them the body they
wanted. I tried. I was always trying.

For the most part I found potential suitors on the Internet. And
that's where I met Roy. Based on his dating profile, WriterRoy was my
male doppelgänger. He was a writer, getting his master's degree at NYU,
working as a personal trainer to put himself through school. He wanted
to write children's books when he graduated. While I cobbled together a
living as a writer too, my goals weren't quite as saccharine or ambitious.
Writing wasn't my dream—acting was—but I could eat a lot more carbs
as a writer, and I got paid regularly, and those were good enough reasons
as any to gradually segue from acting part-time while holding down a
day job to writing full time. I did mostly fitness-related articles, but I
had a daily gig writing gossip for a major news network. I also worked
as a spin instructor a few days a week for fun/mandatory calorie burn.
I wanted to get my personal-training certificate and maybe a degree
in nutrition somewhere down the line. As Roy and I IM'd about our
mutual interests, I imagined us having a whole life of talking about
word counts and hip adductors.

Despite how perfect he seemed for me, there were some things
about him, things that made me uneasy. For starters he was beautiful:

stammering-and-snorting-at-jokes-uncontrollably-in-his-presence kind of beautiful. Tall, but not so tall that I couldn't reach his lips if I wanted to, lips that were centered in a perfectly square jaw. Olive skin, thick brown hair just a smidge lighter than black. His body was flawless, the hint of his muscular chest and abs evident through his clothes, the fabric taut against his well-developed arms. How attractive he was made me suspicious—why would someone who looked like him want to be with someone who looked like me?

It's not that I thought I was unattractive; I just peaked at cute. Men who looked like Roy should be with sexy women, models. Tall, leggy women with alluring accents and designer clothes. And, from what I could tell, those were the kinds of girls he normally dated.

I'd had a friend who had a job at a dating site keeping up a fake "perfect girl" profile to keep male subscribers paying up each month, so I wasn't completely sure that his online dating profile was genuine when he messaged me for the first time. His profile was a little too flawless to be real.

After a week of e-flirting he friended me on social media in what I assumed was an attempt to see more photos of me. I returned the favor. What became obvious to me even before meeting this tall, dark, Middle Eastern Ken doll was that he was indeed a real person. And he was a player.

There for all the Internet to see were his red flags: very recent photos of him surrounded by swarms of what had to be models and dancers in bikinis at high-profile pool parties and "naked body painting" parties (the kinds of events I would rather be stoned to death than go to), pictures of him and an Australian makeup artist he had briefly dated while she was in town for Fashion Week seeing the sights of New York together, and flirty wall posts from far more outgoing women than I would ever be writing the sorts of things I blushed just reading.

And he was Israeli. I didn't know what it was about Israelis I was so attracted to, but my dating history since Paul had been bordering on fetishistic. I'd even deduced through Facebook that I'd briefly dated someone Roy had gone to high school with in Tel Aviv.

And then there was the disappointment on his face when he saw me the first time. He was surprised by what I really looked like. He explained his disappointed glare when I asked him—I thought I'd done a fairly good job of presenting myself accurately on my profile. "In pictures your hair looks darker; I didn't expect you to be so blonde."

I'd never met a man who was upset about me being blonde. I knew that wasn't it. He hadn't expected me to be quite so not thin. I was actually in a thin-for-me phase, one of the rare moments in my adulthood that I'd managed to keep my BMI in the normal weight category—but I was fleshy, curvy with thick hips and thighs. I didn't look like the girls he usually surrounded himself with.

I knew that before he did and had kept putting off our first date in an attempt to lose a few pounds. I told him my dance card was full, that I had work commitments, that I was visiting my family, all the while skipping meals and showing his picture to my friends for advice.

I'd downloaded photos of him from Facebook and promptly sent them to my closest friends, even my parents.

"He's too attractive to date, right?"

My father said he looked like he'd been Photoshopped, and my mother downloaded a topless photo of him to her computer just for fun and started referring to him as "Abs." If our date didn't go well, she could at the very least send his photo to her friends for a little eye candy and gossip. My friends said, "He's attractive . . ." Some followed up with "See how it goes." Others were more complimentary.

"Kim, you're beautiful," my friend Becky IM'd me back. Since she was an attorney who spent a good deal of her time securing restraining orders against the abusive husbands of her clients, I knew she had better things to do with her time than coddle my ego, but I still felt the need to bother her at work.

"You have the most well-proportioned face I have ever seen," she typed at me.

I wasn't self-conscious about my face, and that was a weird compliment, but I took it because I needed it.

I wasn't just fishing for compliments. I was asking if Roy was *too* attractive to be kind and loyal, to not use me or hurt me. I knew those things aren't mutually exclusive, but I also knew that the world treated beautiful people differently. They were forgiven, even expected to have a certain amount of misbehavior.

I just didn't want to be on the receiving end of that behavior again. I was so tired of trying, so tired of putting myself out there only to be told that I'm great but not quite what anyone wanted. I had thought I would marry Paul, but that hadn't worked out.

Dating is a numbers game, I told myself every single time I logged in to JDate or OKCupid, but it was one I was weary of playing. In the three years since Paul, I got really good at giving and receiving the "You're great, but . . ." speech. *That,* that right there, that's what I liked about the Israelis I'd dated: they didn't even lead with a compliment. It was all so straightforward with them; if they wanted to have casual sex with you, they'd tell you; if they wanted to marry you, they'd tell you; if you weren't doing it for them, they'd tell you that too. Nothing personal. "I just don't want you."

I put off meeting him for weeks, but Roy was persistent and I was curious. When I couldn't avoid him anymore, I agreed to meet him for a quick, noncommittal bite to eat on a Monday afternoon in July. He was off from school, and my daily gossip deadline was sometime before the break of dawn, leaving me to roam the city freely while everyone else was at work. After his initial look of disappointment, I wrote him off completely. *Just get through lunch,* I told myself as we walked from Union Square's iconic statue of George Washington atop his steed to a nearby Thai restaurant—President Washington and I both a little battle worn.

At first the conversation was banal. He asked me about my career as a writer, and I thought he was fishing for me to connect him with my agent. I told him I worked mostly as a freelancer, writing about gossip and fitness for a variety of magazines and websites, and that I had been writing a series of essays, not to publish, maybe to publish—I might show them to my agent eventually—I didn't know.

He asked what they were about and I told him. They were about my past.

"What about your past?"

"Well, I'm writing about my family—my dad has an obsessive-compulsive disorder." That wasn't completely true; the DSM-5 had recently relabeled hoarding as its own disorder, but that was far too complicated to explain on a first date.

"Does he wash his hands a lot?"

"No." I wasn't sure I wanted to tell him this, but I was fairly confident I'd never see him again. "He's a hoarder."

Roy was remarkably unfazed by my confession, and I wondered if maybe he didn't understand what I was saying. He certainly didn't understand the breadth of baggage I carried. Instead of acknowledging my deepest, darkest secret, he asked for the check and took me to the Strand, a bookstore in the East Village, so that we could talk about what kinds of books we liked.

As we roamed the graphic-novel shelves, I realized that he was a geek: a beautiful Superman-loving, Captain America–worshipping comic-book geek—and I started to relax a little. After books we had ice cream, and after ice cream we had coffee until it was six p.m. and I had to go to a writing class and he had to go train a client.

On the corner of Eighteenth Street and Fifth Avenue, I kissed him on the cheek and walked away, willing myself not to look back. That had gone a lot better than I'd expected.

I was excited, but that didn't stop me from trying to break things off with him date after date—I couldn't get past his initial look of disappointment. He told me he wanted to change my mind about him. He called when he said he would, texted me daily to say he was thinking of me, and never let more than two days pass without planning a date.

How attentive he was being was novel and a little alarming. I had never been treated that way.

"Dad, what does it mean if a guy calls you every day? That's weird, right?" I was home for the weekend, and as if I were fourteen years old again, the only thing I could bring myself to talk about was the boy I liked. But as far as my go-to for the male perspective, I had to ask my dad for advice—he is brutally honest about everything.

"It means he's controlling," my mother chimed in from the kitchen, but my father waved her comment away with his hand.

"Let's see," my dad said, looking at the newspaper for answers. "Either he likes you or he hasn't gotten laid in a while."

I was pretty sure it wasn't the latter. Based on his social media account, Roy had no problem getting laid. I decided I would give this man—who seemed so honestly smitten with me—a real shot.

One month after our first date Roy and I went to a café on the Upper West Side, an Israeli chain of cafés with an Italian name. Over a dinner of salads and shakshuka, he presented me with a toothbrush and asked me if I would be his girlfriend, officially.

I hadn't been a girlfriend in a long time. But I wanted to be. We were already spending most nights together—since I lived in Brooklyn and he on the Upper West Side, it was basically a long-distance relationship, and staying over was always easier than taking the long train ride home at the end of the night. And, well, I wanted to be with him all the time. I said yes.

One evening while he was out training and I was left behind in his Cold War–era bomb-shelter-turned-studio-apartment, I decided to use his computer to get a head start on the gossip articles I had due in the morning.

I was searching for dirt on a since-forgotten reality TV star when my insecurities took over. There, on his computer with access to his social media and email accounts, I started searching for anything he had confessed to friends about me. It didn't take long for the email to come up. He had written to a friend about me a week or so before, a set designer whom he had trained years earlier at one of Chelsea's prime gay gyms (New York has niche everything).

> On the other hand, she has a big butt and a belly, which bother me, and as you said, it's likely to only get worse. So I'm not sure what I want to do . . .

His friend's response was that he needed to get out immediately, because if I was chunky now, I'd always be chunky, and he'd end up miserable with a fatty and ultimately screw me up for life.

Little did he know that I'd already had a lifetime of being screwed up for life.

THE BIRTH AND DEATH OF BODY ACCEPTANCE

It was purple satin and had "Diary" embossed in gold thread across the cover. A copper lock gave the illusion of privacy, but I didn't need (or want) much privacy in the third grade. I wrote each entry in my first diary as if it were a letter to a future biographer, imagining that one day I would be famous and long after I died the journals of my youth would be sold at auction or displayed in a museum.

The therapist I saw after our house had burned down had recommended the journal as a therapeutic tool so that I could reflect on my family's loss privately, but I never wrote about the fire or mourning my pets, about leaving my friends, or the less-than-stellar adjustment I was making at my new school. I didn't write about how our new house had started to fill up with the same clutter we'd escaped in our old house or my parents fighting. Writing things down made them permanent, and I didn't want history to reflect any of it. My future readers would only know me as a success story, and so night after night I wrote about my plans to be a famous Broadway actress and all the ways I planned on losing weight in preparation.

It didn't take long until I'd filled up the small purple diary with my carefully concocted plans to cut calories, take more dance classes, and do more crunches. That diary was eventually traded in for one adorned with Raphael's cherubs, and after that, one boasting a quote by Eleanor Roosevelt, and eventually a series of marbled composition books. I kept writing in my diaries until I left for college, lugging with me a decade of dietary confessions to Boston, then Los Angeles, and finally to my Brooklyn apartment. I threw them out one day during a cleaning binge. I didn't open them. I didn't have to; I knew what they said. Twenty years later my journal entries and priorities hadn't changed all that much. If I could find a way to weigh absolutely nothing, then I might be happy.

Social historian and professor emerita of Cornell University Joan Jacobs Brumberg spent years collecting the journals of adolescent girls from throughout the last century, and she documented the commonalities and differences in the experiences of young women in her book *The Body Project*. She went so far as to put ads in the newspaper requesting people donate any adolescent journals they might have in their possession. I thought about sending her my old diaries, but I assumed her research was over and felt that my own adolescent ramblings were both abhorrently uninteresting and atrociously spelled.

Early in *The Body Project* she contrasts two diary entries from girls about the same age, making New Year's resolutions ninety years apart:

In 1892, the New Year's resolutions of an adolescent girl were that she was "resolved, not to talk about myself or feelings. To think before speaking. To work seriously. To be self-restrained in conversation and actions. Not to let my thoughts wander. To be dignified. Interest myself more in others."

Fast forward to the year I was born, 1982: "I will try to make myself better in any way I possibly can with the help of my budget and babysitting money. I will lose weight, get new lenses, already got new haircut, good makeup, new clothes, and accessories."

The century between these two new years marked an important shift in how Americans prioritized their body image, one that neither of those young women probably understood in their time.

The industrial revolution that spanned the mid-eighteenth and nineteenth centuries created more jobs and a growing middle class, and with it more disposable income and exposure to entertainment, especially among women who were entering the workforce in droves. Women's media—even then—emphasized the importance of fashion, and with that, there was a new pressure for women to have the perfect body. Very, very thin.

It has been theorized that a root of the frail, delicate ideals of female beauty in the Victorian era can be traced back to *Pamela* by Samuel Richardson, an eighteenth-century bestseller whose popularity at the time rivaled that of the *Twilight* saga today. The heroine of the novel is a young (fifteen-year-old) serving maid who writes to her family of her employer's ardent attempts to "seduce" her (with rape), but she holds her ground and her virtue, and he eventually stops trying to stick his penis in her unwilling vagina and decides that a better way to get her into bed would be to offer her the holy bonds of matrimony, thus elevating her from her lowly origins to the life of aristocracy she deserves for being small, and frail, and always honorable. Tiny, pale, and pious, just like Pamela, became ideals to which women of any class could and should aspire. Corsets, an undergarment designed to minimize a woman's waist while accentuating her bust and hips, had already been around for centuries, but by the time the Victorian era dawned, corset fashion demanded that the wearer constrain her waist to an optimal eighteen inches—akin to that of a toddler—while the skirt below ranged from hoop skirt to form-fitting bustle meant to exaggerate her hip-to-waist or hip-to-buttocks ratios.

Author Lois Banner writes of the era in her book *American Beauty*, "Small hands and feet had long been considered a mark of nobility. Slim waists were the luxury of a social class that did not have to live on a heavy starch diet. Small noses and mouths too were seen as signs of superior gentility, as was a pale complexion." In the early to mid-nineteenth century, women, at least rich women, were at their most beautiful when they were considered childlike.[1]

While the ladies of wealth and breeding spent their days studying people who were ill in order to take on a more fragile demeanor themselves, the United States was seeing a more robust body type emerge with the influx of poor German immigrants. A peasant class, usually farming families, came to the United States in droves and brought with them their voluptuous, uncorseted physiques. By the mid-nineteenth century, curves had gained popularity in the entertainment industry (which in its early days primarily catered to the immigrant population), and by the height of the vaudeville era, in the mid to late nineteenth century, society had started to favor heavier frames. To keep up with the fashion, women who had once aspired to a waist comparable to that of a small child started putting on twenty, thirty, forty, or more pounds to fit a new standard of beauty.

The age of the fleshy woman was short lived. By the late nineteenth century and early twentieth century, there was a new body type to strive for, and women were back on a diet. Bland vegetarian diets became the rage among the socially Christian crowd, as did the sallow looks

---

1.   In that sense, not much has changed. A 2004 Finnish study published in *The American Journal of Public Health* found a clear correlation between income and weight, with those of higher income weighing significantly less than those of lower income, most likely because they have better nutrition education and access to healthier food.

they often resulted in,[2] thanks to Sylvester Graham and John Harvey Kellogg, while Horace Fletcher, "the Great Masticator," spread his belief that food should be chewed about one hundred times per minute before being swallowed. Depending on the composition of the food, that is—a shallot, he suggested, should be chewed seven hundred times before swallowing. Some of his famous followers included Henry James, Franz Kafka, and the US military—the US government experimented with having soldiers chew their food for extensive periods of time in hopes that the practice would cut down on food costs. They were right: it took so long for troops to finish their meals that their meal breaks were over before they could go back for seconds.

By the turn of the twentieth century, the American public had agreed upon a new ideal female body, and it wasn't based on a book or emulating voluptuous entertainers or an exotic new immigrant population—it was based on a drawing. The Gibson girl, drawn for *Life* magazine in the 1890s by Charles Dana Gibson, became an unlikely standard of beauty toward the end of the century. Tall and lean with an ample bosom, the Gibson girl was educated and independent, but not too independent, an everywoman and an ideal woman in one. She became a phenomenon, and drawings of her became the standard to which real-life women strove. The Gibson girl was tall, thin, and athletically built, naturally. Dieting wouldn't become a national pastime for Americans again until the onset of World War I.

By the time World War I started, Americans had just come from a century of losing and gaining and losing and gaining weight. The calorie had been "debuted" to the weight-concerned public in 1894 (although it had been acknowledged scientifically since 1848); the first diet book had been written (see Banting, page 43); a booming industry of diet

---

2.   I'm not suggesting that vegetarian diets in general lead to an emaciated appearance; it was the low-in-fat-and-protein diets that Graham and Kellogg promoted that tended to lead to this particular result.

gurus was emerging. Still, the majority of people were more focused on getting enough to eat than on dieting. Losing weight was a luxury for people who could afford to need to, but when a war broke out in Europe, the government made reducing your food portions and your waistline an act of patriotism.

In her book *The Hundred Year Diet*, Susan Yager writes of the government's promotion of dieting as a means of being patriotic. A young Herbert Hoover, at the time the federal food administrator, encouraged the American public to restrict their own eating so that there would be enough food to send to the armed forces. "Do Not Help the Hun at Meal Time" banners hung proudly all over the country as a not-so-subtle reminder that by eating too much, a patriotic American was inadvertently aiding the enemy.

Losing weight became a national form of entertainment. Newspapers hosted *Biggest Loser*–style weight-loss competitions with dueling "health expert" coaching teams, fans catching up with their favorite contestants' results in the Sunday paper each week. Having a personal scale at home became a status symbol, as knowing how much you weighed at all times of the day became of vital importance. Those who couldn't afford a scale (at the hefty price of $12.95, or the equivalent of $180.20 today) could use public penny scales. And they did—in full force. In 1927 the newly weight-obsessed public spent more than $5 million to weigh themselves, the equivalent of $68.1 million today.

Quickly moving from a sickly look to a stockier size to a Gibson girl, only six short decades had passed before being overweight was downright un-American—it became perfectly acceptable to berate a person for their lack of thinness.

We never stood a chance.

By 1982, when an anonymous everygirl was resolving to use all her babysitting money to better herself by bettering her appearance, dieting had transitioned from a once-taboo task taken on by an unfortunate but prosperous few to a socially expected habitude. By the time I started college, I had been on Jenny Craig, Weight Watchers, some bizarre diet Suzanne Somers had come up with that was a lot like keeping kosher, Atkins, and Stillman; went long periods without eating more than five hundred calories a day; and spent a summer at fat camp. And I wasn't alone; my friends and I would often undertake diet-of-the-day challenges together, hoping that peer pressure would be enough to shame us into prolonged good behavior.

There isn't a single chapter of my life where I wasn't following some type of diet—except for two outlying periods when I allowed myself to exist in the world without a diet to organize my days around. The first was when I was eighteen and studying abroad in the Netherlands my sophomore year of college. I spent the better part of 2001 eating crusty white breads with hunks of cheese, drinking coffee with real sugar, dipping warm chips in mayonnaise, and sipping tepid beer at the pub frequented by the middle-class Dutch families that lived in the town and the college sophomores who had invaded it. I lost fifteen pounds. I didn't know I'd lost weight—the castle I lived in didn't have a scale—but when I went to meet my parents at the airport on the way home, my mother walked right past me. She didn't recognize me.

It was a fluke, I told myself, crediting the weight loss with less processed "European food." In America I still needed to diet. As soon as I was back on campus I went back to Weight Watchers and the eighteen points a day I was allowed to eat. The plan changed every year or so, but my weight didn't. One week I'd lose a pound; the next I'd gain it back and berate myself for being the same weight I always was. The cashier told me I could change my goal weight so I could become a lifetime member and stop paying, but I needed the ten-dollar-a-week investment in potential public shaming. If I were to allow myself to fictitiously reach my goal, then I might make maintenance a reality and never be as thin as I needed to be. The act of standing in a long line of women waiting patiently to be ushered onto the scale by a stranger once a week was what I needed to keep me from going out to dinner with friends or sleeping through my five a.m. gym alarm. I counted points right up until the day Paul and I broke up, and then I stopped. It didn't matter that I'd spent years becoming a polyglot in the world of invented food linguistics; I'd failed to be perfect enough to be deserving of love or loyalty, so what good was it?

After Paul left I ate all the things, my second period of untracked consumption, rebellion against all the years of carefully planned meals and deprivation that was supposed to shield me from failure and disappointment. I checked off each item on my "never allowed" list in a mission to somehow get back at Paul for sleeping with someone thinner. I ordered takeout for the first time in my adult life and skipped the gym because I didn't want to run into him in the weight room. I gained thirty pounds. Quickly. Uncomfortably. I hated myself, but that was nothing new. I hid myself away from the world, avoiding social events and backing out of auditions. I didn't want anyone to see me the way I really was.

I diverted all the attention I'd spent on auditions and exercise to the LSATs. Instead of rehearsals, I spent my weekends going on tours of law schools. I wasn't completely sure I wanted to be a lawyer, but I wanted to go back to school, to do something normal, grounded people did. I wanted to get away from the city and industry I shared with Paul. I liked the idea of spending my days behind a desk in an air-conditioned office. I didn't have to be an actor, someone who was constantly struggling to be funny enough, flirty enough, pretty enough, someone whose weight was a commodity to be hired and fired by; I could just be a normal person who was allowed to be imperfect.

When my acceptance letters started to roll in, I wasn't excited, but I was resolved to trying out a completely different life. I just had one last audition to go to before I decided where to spend the next three years. I'd seen a casting notice for an online talk show, produced by an unnamed magazine publishing company. They wanted a comedic actress with an interest in health and fitness, but there was one noteworthy prerequisite: she needed to be a size ten or higher. And it was paid. It was too good not to submit for, even though I knew my acting days were behind me.

I submitted my headshot, assuring them that I wasn't nearly as slender as I looked in my photos (a first!), and a few weeks later got a call to come in to audition.

The studio was a few blocks from my Park Slope apartment, an industrial complex near the Gowanus Canal that had been converted into artists' studios. Within a few years this area would welcome posh bars and boutiques, a Whole Foods Market, and apartment complexes that only the Wall Street elite could afford, but at the time it was still littered with trash and needles and more than a few "ladies of the night," as my father often referred to the women who worked the area, regardless of the time of day.

Jenn, the production intern, met me at the door to the building and led me to an unpainted, unfurnished, unventilated room with a tripod. My screen test consisted of answering a few questions about how I like my ice cream and five minutes of a stand-up routine I'd been asked to prepare about a new exercise trend: naked yoga. It was supposed to be funny, but I was betraying the set of rules I live by: never admit you're fat. I wasn't supposed to eat ice cream, never mind like it or talk about liking it. And I definitely wasn't supposed to acknowledge the paranoia that accompanied each trip to the gym—even in clothes—that others might be thinking the exact same things about my body that I was. Making jokes about my body meant being laughed at for my body, and I wasn't sure I was strong enough to do that.

It was hot, probably in the low nineties outside, but the airless warehouse-turned-audition-space was easily a hundred degrees, and I'd decided to wear the only top that minimized my new thirty pounds: a sweater. I joked and sweated and delivered my naked-yoga routine to the red flashing light in front of me, hoping desperately for a chuckle or grin from Jenn, something, anything that might indicate I was funny and not just a caricature.

And that was it. No laughs, just a face full of caking makeup that was starting to itch and an unpaid intern thanking me for my time.

I got a call from the show's director, Sebastian, the next day. He wanted me to come back, to write another routine about diet and fitness and perform for him in his (thankfully air-conditioned) office.

It was the same dilapidated building, but the production office had windows and air and people wearing headphones who lined the walls working from giant Mac screens on animation or editing already-filmed clips of shows I would have nothing to do with. There was even an Emmy—a real one, not the kind you pick up on Hollywood studio tours—sitting on one of the shelves, being used as a bookend. Casual, no big deal, just an Emmy.

"Hi, Kimberly, I'm Sebastian. I loved your first tape," he greeted me when I walked in the door. First impression: he looked like LA, or at least how I imagined an LA director looked. Thin and angular, with tight jeans and a button-down shirt unbuttoned at the top and untucked at the bottom. He told me about his history as an animator (which was what he won the Emmy for), the new production company he'd launched with his brother, and this mysterious project I'd been called in for.

Condé Nast was producing a new blog network made up of three sites: Daily Bedpost, about sex and relationships and tied to *Glamour*; Product Fiend, a makeup site connected to *Allure*; and Elastic Waist, which would be under the *Self* umbrella. The secret project was for the Elastic Waist show. They were looking to expand in new forms of media—now that they'd had some great bloggers on board—and wanted someone to host a daily web show reflecting current weight-loss trends and gimmicks.

As he told me about the site's niche market of women who loved health and fitness but who were fed up with the diet industry and being told constantly that they'd never be good enough because they just weren't built that way or refused to live a life devoid of culinary pleasures, I realized that there were other options. I'd never heard of the fat-acceptance movement or body positivity or health at any size, but I liked the idea that there were people out there who believed in this. I wanted to know these people, to be like these people. If size acceptance was a religion, I was ready to be converted.

I didn't have to go back into the unventilated room this time; I set up shop in the middle of the production office and did my stand-up in front of the editors, animators, and interns. And I was nervous; whatever this was, I wanted to be a part of it. I didn't want to be a lawyer. I wanted to be the poster girl for a movement I'd never heard of.

And I was. The call came a few days later. The *Devil Wears Prada* crowd I imagined in the Condé Nast building had chosen me.

I deferred law school in favor of four a.m. joke-writing sessions—jokes that wouldn't be at my expense or the expense of the bodies of the people who watched the show, but of society, of ad campaigns and diet trends—and for six a.m. call times on set. Afterward I would race to work as a fundraiser for a national nonprofit, then after work I would head out for auditions, shows, and rehearsals. My new schedule changed everything about how I ate; my focus shifted from wanting to be thin (because for the first time I didn't *have* to be) but simply surviving my schedule. Instead of counting calories, I focused on eating for optimal energy—I didn't really have a game plan; I just tried to eat the foods that made me feel good physically and kept me awake during my very long days. Within six months of starting my web series *The Daily Special*, I had gone from a size twelve back to a size eight, and it had been effortless. I decided right then and there that I had found the secret; the key to being thin was being busy and happy. That was it, I thought. I just had to be busy and happy all the time and I would stay thin.

Simple. Except my weight loss was a problem. One of my job requirements was that I be at least a size ten. I opened every email my producer sent me with trepidation, but the ruling class in the Times Square HQ liked my progression, and they wanted me to work my weight loss into the show. It was a different angle; we could show people that being body positive didn't mean not wanting to lose weight if that's what you wanted, but loving yourself no matter what.

Self magazine ran an annual diet series, "The Self Challenge," and it was the perfect opportunity to brown nose the mothership. I followed the twelve-week magazine diet as best I could and blogged about it in what was supposed to be a short-lived blog called *The Kim Challenge*—I didn't care about the diet; I just wanted to keep my job and hoped that the producers might notice me as a writer. I took pictures of everything I ate on the diet and wrote about my exercise and weight loss. When the twelve weeks were over, readers wrote to me and asked me to keep it up, so I did (going on nine years). Most importantly, the powers that be at Condé Nast noticed and asked me to start writing for their blog network.

I was a master at passive-aggressive self-promotion. And now I was a writer.

I kept writing my personal blog in addition to my new daily column on Elastic Waist. And I bought it, hook, line, and sinker. I was a believer; we're all in this together. Every time I sat down at my computer to work on my post for the day, I opened a new vein of insecurity, and the strangers on the other side of my words wrote back that they understood. I was never going to get rid of my "fat pants" or my "skinny jeans"—I knew from experience that I'd need them both again at some point. I had never had a problem talking about my diet of the day to anyone who asked, because being on a diet meant that I was trying, but I'd never actually admitted how much my weight consumed me, how it had dictated every decision I made. People I didn't know wrote to me regularly to tell me they felt the exact same way. It didn't matter what their actual weight was or where they fell on the BMI chart; they never felt like they were small enough or good enough. It wasn't just me—it was everyone. Maybe not *everyone*, but a good portion of everyone.

I was flying high on a sense of solidarity when I decided to make my "fat pic" public.

It was my shameful secret: proof of my failure, my rock bottom. I'd kept it in my wallet since I graduated from high school. I'd spent years stroking it while in line for weigh-in, or as motivation to order a salad instead of a sandwich or to never, ever skip a cardio session.

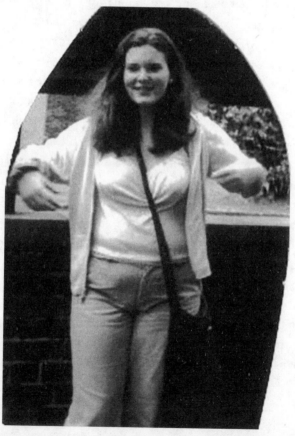

I usually threw out bad photos of me, but there was something about this picture. I put it in my wallet, a reminder of what I never wanted to look like again.

I look happy enough in it, but then again, I always looked happiest when life was hardest. By the time my senior year had started, my father's hoarding had reached an unlivable level of squalor. Our house had started to fall apart around us: first leaky pipes made the whole house damp and smell like mildew, then a broken boiler meant no hot water for showers and no heat in the winter, and eventually a collapsed ceiling in our kitchen rendered it completely useless. We figured out ways to get around it. We joined a gym and showered there. We bought space heaters for our bedrooms and a mini fridge and microwave for the upstairs. We existed on fast food and snack cakes that can live forever in cellophane. My weight skyrocketed, but I didn't know how to stop it; I didn't have any options. I'd stopped weighing myself after I hit 188 pounds, after someone had taken a picture of me posing in front of a museum, sopping wet from rain. My wet tank top clung to my body, accentuating my bloated breasts and stomach. My stomach formed a perfect "8," round everywhere except where my too-tight pants pulled my stomach in; my face, a perfect circle. I usually threw out bad photos of me, but there was something about that picture. I put it in my wallet, a reminder of what I never wanted to look like again. I took it with me everywhere. I just wanted to go to college and start over. I'd lose weight then, when I could eat normal food.

And I did. Breakfast cereals, salads, and sandwiches: the cafeteria was full of normal food, and by the end of my freshman year I had returned to somewhere in the high 140s, which seemed to be my body's set point. I may have been the only person in the history of college to lose the freshman forty. I kept that picture of myself in my wallet for years so that I would always remember what I looked like at almost 190 pounds.

***

The readers of Elastic Waist were my safe zone, a place where I could write about wanting to allow that girl to rest in peace instead of holding her up on a pedestal by which I could constantly torment myself.

After I posted my fat pic, the backlash was immediate. I'd never had so many comments on a post. While some people thought I was brave to post a picture of myself at my least confident on the Internet, the majority told me I was nothing but an attention whore, a fat shamer. My photo was "hurtful" to people who had never been as thin as I was in my fat picture. Even though my BMI put me in the obese category, I wasn't "fat enough" to have a fat picture. I was only perpetuating the societal expectations that Elastic Waist had been a respite from.

When my blog was syndicated on other sites, the comment sections were littered with anonymous critiques of my fat physique, but my "friends" on Elastic Waist thought I was mocking them. There was a hierarchy that I was realizing I didn't fit into: I wouldn't ever be thin enough to be thin enough and I didn't weigh enough to have an acceptable place in the size-acceptance movement.

The show was canceled in 2008 when the economy crashed. A few days later the nonprofit I worked for laid off the majority of the New York office. I very literally had nothing to do. So I went back to acting, and all the body confidence I had learned over the almost two years I taped *The Daily Special* vanished overnight.

CANADIAN PILL PUSHERS

The veneration of the superficial isn't something we invented in the twentieth century. As long as we've lived within the confines of society, humans have found a standard of beauty to lust after and aspire to, be it the long, lean limbs of Nefertiti in fourteenth-century BCE Egypt; the muscular preferences of the ancient Greeks,[1] the predilection for pale, slightly built bodies in the Han Dynasty, or the full hips and breasts and pale skin ubiquitous to Renaissance art.

Darwin called it aesthetic evolution, and it was considered one of his most controversial ideas, in that it suggests we use sexual selection to mate for beauty. Naysayers of aesthetic evolution suggested that the idea of mating for beauty would put the gene pool at risk because it emphasizes traits that are not useful for survival over ones that are. But as someone who found her mate on the Internet by browsing photos accompanied by lists of academic accolades and tax-bracket statuses, I see it alive and well in how we as a species choose to evolve from here on out.

---

1.   Aristotle called the female form "a deformed male."

Nature has a way of sorting these things out. The castle I lived in in the Netherlands doubled as a dorm and bird sanctuary. The only species that seemed to know that they had found a safe haven were peafowl. Peacocks have evolved intricate plumes as a way of attracting hens; the more colorful the plume, the more likely they were to reproduce. But because vibrant color will also attract predators, there's a good chance that the prettiest peacock also has stellar survival skills, increased speed, and strength. With pretty, pretty peacocks getting their pick of the peahen crop to breed with, eventually the number of pretty peacocks would increase, tipping the genetic scale in their favor.

Peafowl are not indigenous to America,[2] but the appreciation and expectation of a fine physique is as American as apple pie. When founding father Alexander Hamilton wrote to his friend John Laurens in 1779 requesting help finding a wife, his list of must-haves started with "She must be young—handsome (I lay most stress upon a good shape)." He ended up marrying Elizabeth Schuyler, a socialite and daughter of a Revolutionary War general. The paintings that survive of her show her to be pale and slim, albeit corseted, as was the fashion of the time. She may not have actually fit the ideal body of her time, which was much heavier—disease was rampant in colonial America, and women with fuller builds were considered healthier, more likely to withstand the harsh living that was eighteenth-century America.[3]

---

2. But turkeys are.

3. Our forefathers and mothers may have been onto something; a 2009 study published in *The Journal of the American Medical Association* found that those with a BMI in the overweight range, twenty-five to thirty, had a 6 percent lower risk of death (in any given period) than people whose BMI fit in what is considered the normal range (18.5 to 25). The researchers from the CDC, who analyzed ninety-seven studies and 2.88 million people worldwide, found that these percentages were consistent globally and within all age groups. They did, however, find that the risk of death increased once the BMI escalated above thirty-five, which would be considered squarely in the obese range.

By the twenty-first century the body types our foreparents coveted for their hardiness became a health crisis in and of themselves. Two-thirds of Americans are now considered overweight, and achieving status in the remaining under- to normal-weighted third has become an industry that rivals (and outperforms) the GDP of many countries—an industry I had inadvertently found myself a part of as I transitioned my blog-a-day stint of writing about my bodily insecurities into the world of fitness magazines. But while I worked on figuring out how to have a writing career, I was also left deciding if I still wanted an acting one.

After *The Daily Special* was canceled, my performing opportunities became less and less frequent. I had a bit part in an indie film that did well on the festival circuit and still performed at storytelling events and improv comedy shows around the city, but I wasn't sure what place there was for me in the real scripted-acting world anymore. At twenty-seven, I wasn't exactly a "hot young thing." I'd been cast mostly as naive ingénues in my early twenties, but now there were new girls in their early twenties who were getting those roles. I wasn't particularly quirky, and I couldn't yet pass for mom roles. It seemed like my little web series that made fun of society's ridiculous standards had been the zenith of my acting career. I wasn't being fatalistic—that was about as much as I could expect from my acting degree.

Eight months passed between when *The Daily Special* was canceled and when I got my next "acting" gig. I wasn't busy or happy anymore. I wasn't even thirty, but I was pretty sure I'd achieved has-been status.

When my commercial agent's number showed up on my caller ID, I assumed it was a regular check-in about my measurements. I always lied, but even my lies changed sizes on a regular basis, always within the vicinity of what I could lose in a couple of weeks plus Spanx. It really didn't matter; he never sent me out anyway. I was basically a client in clerical responsibilities only.

"Kimberleeeey." It was actually my agent, not his assistant. "I got a call for you. It's some diet thing. I'm not really sure; I didn't submit you for it . . ."

It wasn't unheard of to be called in for something randomly; the casting director may have used me before, or they may have my head-shot on file for something else I had been submitted but not called in for. I'd never auditioned for a diet product before, which meant there was probably a casting director out there that thought they were doing me a solid, maybe someone who watched my web show or read my weekly fitness column on *Social Workout*. My agent didn't care about where this audition came from or who thought I needed to drop a few pounds. He'd still take home 15 percent of whatever I made regardless.

"Do I need to have any sides prepared?"

"No sides, you just need to wear a bikini," he told me before rattling off my time slot and the address of the casting.

I'd only been asked to wear a bathing suit only one other time in my career, and it hadn't ended well. I was eight, and Chickie had sent me out on a call for some sort of Club Med–like resort's commercial—that may or may not have actually been Club Med. If I got the job, my family would get a free vacation; they would fly us all to some tropical location and put us up for the duration of the shoot. I really wanted to go on vacation—my family didn't do vacations regularly—and when we did they were educational: Colonial Williamsburg. Amish Country. The Franklin Institute. I'd never been to a resort.

My father and I had been caught in traffic on the way to the city and were an hour late for my audition—I ran through the lobby, leaving my dad behind as the maintenance staff was shutting down the building's main lights. It was closing time, and I just wanted to smile for the camera before the casting agents left for the day. When the casting agent handed me a navy-blue one-piece, I became shy; no one had mentioned anything about a bathing suit. I didn't think I had an option to say no. In third grade, I was keenly aware of the fact that I was not one of the skinny girls. The casting agent left me alone in her office to change, and I debated wearing my underwear under the suit or not. I knew other girls had been wearing the same bathing suit all day, but I took off my underwear because they added bulk. Every little bit counted.

The casting agent had looked me over and said I could go, just as my father was getting off the elevator to meet me. Nineteen years later, I had a feeling this would be a very similar situation. Still, I needed to pay rent, and my agent called so rarely, I didn't feel like I could say no and stay on his roster.

"What does it pay?" I asked.

"Six thousand dollars. It's a print ad and national commercial run," he told me.

Six thousand dollars isn't much when it comes to national commercials. A good national commercial could buy you a house in some parts of this country (not New York), but I was making a living off freelance writing jobs, which meant living off my credit cards until one of my many employers decided they could pay me.

Six thousand was worth my pride.

For a girl who grew up on an island, I spent a surprising amount of time avoiding any situation that would require me to wear a bathing suit. I had one, somewhere in the recesses of my closet; the last time I could remember wearing a bikini I was twenty and living in Los Angeles. I was thinner then, and had decided to try out a two-piece for the first time. I tried on dozens, until I finally found one that didn't cut into the fleshy part of my hips: in a moment of genius or desperation, I wandered over to the maternity rack at the Gap. The maternity bikini was my dirty little secret. I'd never been pregnant, but I could see that the maternity bikinis were cut a bit wider on the bottom and had thicker straps, generally a more flattering look for someone who happens to carry most of her weight between her hips and thighs. I was embarrassed every single time I wore it, but it served a purpose that the Victoria's Secret catalog couldn't.

I raced home to fish out my abandoned bathing suit, put on some makeup, and pick out a summer dress that could easily be ditched when the disrobing began.

I'd been to just about every rehearsal space in Manhattan, but I didn't know the address of the place I was headed. It was in the right part of town for auditions, but it looked like a run-down office building, making me even more nervous about what I was getting myself into. It was entirely possible that I was walking into a chubby-girl fetish horror movie, which to be honest I would have done gladly if it paid.

My tensions eased a bit when I opened the door and saw a familiar face. I knew the photographer. Noah was a friend, an actor and model, someone I knew from the comedy circuit. Then my tensions returned—this guy was going to see me in a bikini. I worked with him. I saw him regularly and really liked the fact that we had our clothes on 100 percent of those times. Clothes made me slightly less uncomfortable in my skin as a general rule.

Noah looked startled to see me there, but stopped what he was doing and took me aside as soon as I walked in.

"Hey, what are you doing here?" he said while fidgeting with some lights.

"I didn't know you were a photographer," I said back, not answering him.

"Yeah, it pays the rent. Do you want this gig?"

"I don't know. I don't know what it's for."

"Listen, you're perfect for it; I know exactly what they're looking for. Body types like yours, girls with pretty faces who could stand to lose fifteen pounds. Just don't take the pills, okay? You can lose the weight without the pills."

So it was a job for selling diet pills. If you've ever wondered why there was an abundance of minor celebrities shilling diet pills or bus ads boasting easy ways to lose weight, take into account that around 108 million Americans will go on a diet this year—that's a third of the

American population. If you subtract the 22 percent of Americans who are under the age of ten and over the age of seventy—because really you should just get a pass and enjoy yourself at some phases of your life—then you're looking at only slightly less than half of all Americans.

It kind of stung that he admitted so casually that I could lose weight. I knew it, but I preferred to think it was just in my mind. He wasn't wrong, and honestly I needed the six grand. If he could put in a good word for me, I'd take it.

The audition lasted the entire day, consisting of three rounds, and ended up being more like therapy. The first round consisted of an interview where I met one-on-one with a rep from the diet-pill company who happened to be obese. I wasn't judging him for it, but I thought it was a strange representative to send to an audition peddling diet products. Maybe they thought we'd feel more comfortable hanging around in bathing suits with someone else who didn't fit into the societal ideal? The rep asked us why we had gained weight. What he and the company wanted was a good story, something sad and relatable—the kind of story people on their couches at home would nod their head to—yes, that's why they gained weight too. *It wasn't your fault; life handed you an unfair hand; now take these pills and everything will be better.*

But gaining and losing weight was like breathing for me—which was not what they wanted to hear. So instead I told them why I had gained weight most recently.

Shortly after *The Daily Special* ended, my mother had gone into the hospital for a routine gallbladder surgery. The doctor ended up severing the vein going to her liver and, in the process of trying to stop the bleeding, destroyed her bile ducts. By the time they'd been able to stop the bleeding, she'd almost completely bled out, and neither her kidney nor liver functioned on their own anymore. My father had called to tell me that I needed to get home quickly because the doctor said she had a fifty-fifty shot at survival. I spent the next three months with her, existing on hospital food and the treats people made to comfort me. I'd put on weight, about ten pounds; the weight that had come off me so easily while filming *The Daily Special* came back in the hospital cafeteria. I promised the rep and everyone else in the stark white audition room that my mother was doing better now and I was ready to change my life. It was a good sob story.

The rep looked into my eyes and squeezed my hand and confessed that his mother had also been ill recently. He understood. "Why don't you stick around and have your hair and makeup done?"

I'd made it to round two.

As I sat around waiting for the makeup festivities to start, more women just like me were taken behind the curtain to tell their tales of dietary woes. Some would put on their sundresses and leave, some wouldn't, and we'd sit together in our bikinis, all of us trying to find a way to sit that was somehow flattering. All self-conscious arms and legs crossing and uncrossing constantly, nervously, as we acted like the kind of girls who casually hung out in bikinis.

After an hour or so, we were weeded down to five survivors. Noah was right: there was a very specific body type they were looking for. We had different hair colors, different shades of skin, but we were all between five foot three and five foot six, we all looked to be between 150 and 165 pounds, and we all carried our weight in our lower abdomen, hips, and thighs. We were all averagely relatable in our overweight. Our reliable handler assured us that "before and after" ads legally can't be airbrushed.[4] It made sense that the companies who produce them go to great lengths to cast the right people with the right body types: chubby, pear-shaped bodies that would be more likely to sport a small, market-able waist by the time the "after" photo shoot came about.

The makeup guy was sweet, small, and flamboyant. I didn't know him, and we hardly talked, but his gentle touch while curling my hair

---

4. I haven't actually been able to confirm that there's any legal mandate for honesty in regard to the images used in weight-loss product advertising.

and applying eyeliner was comforting and nurturing in a way that a girl in a bikini needs. I wanted to take him home with me so he could give me that girl-next-door-who-actually-knows-how-to-put-on-makeup glow every day. After we'd all been polished, we posed in front of Noah for some still shots. We then told our stories again, this time to the camera—this would be the story they would want to hear on the commercial. I did my best to pause for dramatic effect, making it known that I was holding back tears. The $120,000 theater degree that I'd be paying off until the day I die had amounted to something. Not much—but something.

As I watched each woman relay her story, I couldn't help but think that we were normal. There were far more women that looked like us out there than who looked like the women at just about every other commercial audition I'd gone on.

Every story was mine at some point or another. There was always a reason to be fat, blame to be placed on genetics, boyfriends, jobs, and traumas. None of us had gained weight because we wanted to. Two-thirds of Americans are overweight, and every one of us feels alone in it.

Besides casual niceties, the other girls and I didn't talk. We were intimate in a way that felt forced. We'd spent the day mostly naked together, sharing our excuses and shame, and we were in competition for something we all only half wanted. Which is why it seemed strange when we were all hired. As our company rep and confidant passed out our contracts, it became clear that it wasn't just us: we were just the New York crew; the production team was headed to Dallas next, then Los Angeles. The company was hedging their bets.

Before we left for the day, feeling a lot less special about ourselves, we were weighed in, had our starting weight announced aloud, and were handed a digital scale, a food scale, and a jug of unmarked pills, with the instructions to meet the nutrition team at a hotel the next day where we would get our official diet-pill model diet.

I wasn't going to get $6,000 for just landing this audition. Not only did I effectively have to lose the forty pounds they assigned me, but I would also need to be chosen for the commercial again, pitted against the other diet success stories. I had to be the last dieter standing.

I'd weighed in at 153 pounds. Losing ten pounds wouldn't be a big deal for me since my body seemed to like to hover in the 140s, but 113 was smaller than I could imagine being—I'd tried my whole life to be that small and could never get there.

Noah gave me a hug when I left and reminded me not to take the pills. "It's just a diet; you don't need them."

He didn't understand, though. I'd been dieting my whole life, and I'd never been as thin as they wanted me to get. I would need pills, lipo, and a personal trainer to hit their goal weight for me.

It was clear as soon as I got to the hotel conference room the next morning, skim-milk iced coffee in hand, that this was a mind game.

This wasn't a rehearsal. We weren't being treated like actors who had been cast for a job—we were lifelong failures about to be saved. The diet-pill mothership would be assigning each of us a "nutrition mentor" who would oversee our weight loss and help us change our lives. Our mentor would come up with a specialized eating and exercise program just for us. All we had to do was follow it and take six pills a day. Every Saturday we had to take new pictures in our bikini-clad selves and send them to an anonymous email address for a veiled company somewhere in Canada. The pictures would include shots of us from the front, side, and back, and one of our scale, with our toes showing, so that we could record our weight.

The other girls and I had spent the whole previous day together without bothering to learn each other's names, but before we left we introduced ourselves, and they hatched plans for creating an email support system for one another. I didn't want to get to know them, though. I just wanted to take my pills and eat my turkey breast. There could be only one winner.

I had spent enough time around fitness magazines to know that nothing in their contents is to be trusted. Of course the ads would be no different. I've seen actresses who make no real effort to hide their eating disorders while shooting a cover give interviews about their love of cooking and obsession with a certain cupcake chain for their feature article. Others who work out religiously, clocking four or five hours of hard work in the gym a day, chalk up their exercise routine as nothing more than taking their dog for long walks through the Hollywood Hills or on the beaches of Malibu. I honestly can't even blame them. I wasn't a particularly successful actress, and my body was still the center of my professional life—I can't even imagine how they felt when every bout of preperiod bloat sent the news cycle into a tailspin of pregnancy rumors. I had a strict no-body-shaming policy when I wrote gossip—other people's bodies were none of my business, no matter how famous they were. My body, however, never received the same level of professional respect. As the rep showed us pictures of former success stories, I wondered if anyone at the fitness magazine I worked at part-time would notice if I showed up in the book one month.

Melanie, my nutrition mentor, emailed me the next morning.

> Kimberly, I am so excited to work with you on this life-changing opportunity. I've attached your initial diet and exercise program. Let me know if you have any questions. I'll be in New York next month and would love to meet with you and see how you're doing!
>
> —Mel

The diet wasn't hard to follow; in fact it was a little too easy: green leafy vegetables, lean proteins, and limited carbohydrates and fats. That was basically how I already ate. And the exercise program was beginner level. I'd already been teaching spin classes for four years and had a writing job that consisted of writing reviews of home-workout programs each week.

Between the "We're here to change your life" and "This is how you do a sit-up" rhetoric, I was feeling a mite condescended to and fairly sure that I wasn't going to be their $6,000 model. But I had nothing better to do, and I'd always wanted to be 113 pounds.

I lost a couple of pounds over the first month, but I wasn't losing what I should—they wanted me to lose two to four pounds a week. Melanie adjusted my required-foods list. She didn't want to tell me how many calories I should eat (for legal reasons I'm sure), so she just suggested I remove a few items from my approved food list to speed things up. First it was one of my allotted servings of carbs for the day, then the one egg yolk a day I was allowed to enjoy.

Feeling as desperate as I did when I decided to try the Stillman diet all those years ago, I didn't listen to Noah: I started popping pills from that giant unmarked jug as soon as I got home from my info session. But first I'd Googled all the ingredients. For the most part they were made up of caffeine and herbs with laxative qualities. They wouldn't kill me. They probably wouldn't make me thinner either, but they would at least keep me awake and help me poop.

Every Saturday I started my day in my bikini, making sure to pee twice before I went on the scale to drain every ounce of excess liquid from my system. First the photos: front, side, back. Then I would dutifully get on the scale. First without my camera, and then with it so that I could report any discrepancy. My weight loss was so minor that every ounce counted. When I went to visit my family for the weekend, I'd take my scale with me. If I had a particularly bad week, I'd ask my mom to stand on the scale, loading her tiny frame with books until she weighed somewhere close to what I was supposed to for that week's weigh-in.

After a couple more months of only minor weight loss, my exercise routine was increased to include seven hours of cardio a week, four hours of running, and three spin classes in addition to the three classes a week that I taught, but those didn't count because I wasn't focused on my own calorie burn. I started adding an extra pill in the morning, then another in the afternoon, making it eight pills a day. I went through so many that I had to ask the company to send me a new tub of pills to help me finish off the trial. As I sat on my couch drinking my morning coffee, taking my caffeine laxatives, and writing my daily column, my heart would race hard and heavy, until I would think for a second, *Maybe I shouldn't be doing this.* But that wasn't a notion I had time for. I couldn't fail at being thin enough again. Not when there was money on the line.

After four months I'd lost eight pounds. I had to admit to myself that I looked pretty good, but pretty good was not what the company was looking for. I was supposed to be twenty pounds thinner by now.

I wrote to Melanie and told her that I just couldn't lose the kind of weight they wanted me to. She wrote saying she understood, this can be a really hard process, but she'd been looking over my food diary and thought that maybe the problem was that I ate mustard and hot sauce with my grilled turkey—those condiments have a lot of sodium.

I knew that mustard and hot sauce had sodium, but I didn't think they had twelve pounds' worth of sodium, and wrote back that I just didn't think I was their girl.

They didn't sue me, which is nice, although they might now. I had lost a dress size and over the next six months was able to lose another two pounds, bringing me to an even ten pounds, back to 143.

It didn't matter professionally: my commercial agent dropped me. The only thing I was good for was the diet commercial "before" photo.

FIGHT OR FLIGHT

If her butt is going to undermine the rest
of your relationship because that's the
way you're wired, judgments of being
infantile and superficial aside, that's the
way it is.

Roy's friend was right; it wasn't ever going to get easier for me—I'd been dieting since I was a child, and even when I was thin for me I never seemed to be thin enough for anyone else—not my boyfriends, not my agents, not the trolls on the Internet, not for diet-pill companies. My weight was the one thing in my life I couldn't overcome. As Roy's friend wrote, very clearly, my butt was going to undermine our relationship. As a size eight, I was probably at the top of my game physically—140 was about as thin as I'd ever been able to get—and it just wasn't good enough.

I didn't confess to being a big-butt-and-bellied snoop when Roy came home. I pretended it was just any other night of new-couple bliss, but I was in fight-or-flight mode. I could break things off with him now and leave him to the models and dancers he preferred, or I could diet harder.

I didn't want to break up with Roy. I liked him, more than I liked anyone in a long time. But I wanted him to like me as I was—that's how romance is supposed to work, right? His email encapsulated everything I'd ever believed about myself: I was almost good enough, if it weren't for my body. And my body was my fault.

I couldn't do Atkins or Dukan[1] or Stillman again. Roy was a vegetarian, and the amount of time I spent at his apartment meant meat would be in short supply. Making a "lifestyle change" was just another way of saying I would be on a very slow diet for the rest of my life. I needed something quick, a diet I could fall in love with and commit myself to completely.

"Is something the matter?" Roy asked as he came home. He'd kissed me hello, and I'd kept it short and peckish instead of the more lingering, naked-inducing kind he'd intended.

"I'm fine. One of the Real Housewives is getting divorced, so I have a lot of work to do," I said. "Actually, I think I'm going to go home; it's going to be a long night of gossip mongering for me."

"Are you sure that's it?"

"Yeah, I need to get something into my editor early for the commute crowd; that's it," I said.

"Do you want to grab something to eat before you go?"

---

1.   A high-protein diet created by French doctor Pierre Dukan. The Dukan Diet rose to fame when it was rumored that Kate Middleton used the plan to prepare for her 2011 nuptials to Prince William, Duke of Cambridge.

"Yeah, let's get something healthy. My best friend is getting married in four months; I want to lose weight for the wedding," I told him. I needed an excuse.

Sometime in the midst of my adolescent parade of diets my mother had said to me, "Kim, you can't change from a place of hate. You can only change yourself if you love yourself."

I kept those words with me for years. They were something to aspire to, but I had never been able to have that happy epiphany that comes at the end of chick-lit novels, the ones where the heroine finally acknowledges her worth and her confidence shines through and the whole world is at her feet. My whole world revolved around a constant effort to be better than I was the day before. Self-acceptance was for people who were done working, and I had so much work to do. One day when I had done everything I needed to do, I would sit back and accept myself; I would love myself then. But now, now I had work to do. I couldn't lose weight because I loved me now, but maybe I could lose weight because I wanted to love Roy.

I packed up the week's worth of clothes I'd left at Roy's apartment and my laptop. I hadn't been home in a while and was looking forward to some time in my own space, with my own food, and my own stuff. Roy carried my bright-pink bag proudly as we made our way to a café near the subway.

"I can help you lose weight if you want; it's kind of what I do," Roy said. Usually, I loved hearing about his clients; he'd shown me pictures of clients he'd helped to lose hundreds of pounds. He had been a big deal in Israel: he had degrees in kinesiology and sports nutrition, wrote a weekly fitness column in the country's largest newspaper, and trained Israeli celebrities and taught at the Wingate Institute, Israel's Sports Medicine and Physiotherapy school, where many of the national sports teams are based. He gave up a successful career at home to come to New York and write books for kids.

My usual awe of his expertise was existing somewhere between my desperate need to not be rejected because of my body and resentment toward his obvious eagerness to help me lose weight. I wanted to tell Roy that I'd snooped through his email and knew that he wasn't quite as attracted to me as he claimed, but that would defeat the purpose. Instead of just being a bit on the chubby side, I'd be crazy *and* a bit on the chubby side. So I told him about my goal to be in the best shape of my life in November, because my best friend was getting married and I wanted to be perfect for her special day.

"I'll ask you what I ask all my clients: How do you plan to do that?" he said while giving his order to the cashier: the Aroma Special Salad, no lettuce, extra cucumbers and tomatoes, no olives, no feta, and an extra hard-boiled egg instead of cheese.

"Feta isn't terribly high in fat; it's only about eighty calories an ounce," I said.

"It's full fat. I don't eat any dairy over 4 percent. What do you want?"

"I'll have the same," I said. "I'll count calories and increase my cardio."

"That's a start. What calories are you aiming for?"

"I'll start around 1,400 and work my way down." That was actually way more than I was planning on eating, but I didn't want him to think I was crazy.

"That's probably too much for you. You're not tall or athletic; you could probably go as low as eight hundred," he said.

He was just as crazy as I was. Eight hundred calories was right in my diet comfort zone: extreme. Still, I felt like we needed a little negotiation. I told him that if I started at eight hundred calories my body would plateau, and I couldn't go much lower than that. It was better to start somewhere near 1,100 calories and work my way down as my weight loss stalled.

He agreed, and we had our first project as a couple: making me the girl I believed he wanted to be with.

We belonged to different gyms, but Roy found a cheap, no-frills gym that we could join together and where he could train me when he was off from school or work.

I started spending two hours every day at the gym, sometimes more. I ate eight hundred calories a day right from the beginning, making sure that the calories I burned in my daily cardio sessions equaled or exceeded the amount of food I ate each day. Instead of meals, I drank vials of liquid protein made from watermelon-flavored beef collagen so that I wouldn't lose too much muscle mass as my body started to break down my tissue for fuel.

It didn't take long for it to become a familiar addiction, a feeling of emptiness that had always been comforting. Feeling physically empty made me feel confident in a way nothing else ever had. And so did the compliments that came with it. When people asked if I was losing weight, I would try to act casually and say, "Maybe a little—I've been superbusy with work." I sounded like every celebrity interview I'd ever made fun of. Going to the gym became a part-time job; I carried my gym bag with me wherever I went and knew exactly where every gym I was a member of was located and what their class schedule was. If I had a few minutes of downtime between jobs or meetings, I went to the gym. If I had the whole day off, I would walk the two miles to the gym and walk back after my two-hour sweat session.

I caught a glance at my body one day while Roy and I were having sex, and for the first time ever, I thought that I looked sexy. It was the only moment in my life, other than the moment in the hotel room before my first and only beauty pageant, that I looked at my body with approval, the outline of my ribs evident through my skin.

On the night of my best friend's wedding, four months after our first date, I was twenty-three pounds thinner; my size six dress needed to be pulled up constantly, because I had been too disbelieving that it actually fit to go down to a four—I was the thinnest I'd ever been as an adult. I weighed the same thing I had when I was eleven.

That was also the night Roy told me he loved me for the first time.

FIFTY POUNDS
TO GALILEE

You can never stop dieting. There's no end—there's just finding a plan of starving yourself that you can live with for the rest of your life. And that's the hard part, figuring out how to not gain weight again.

My first mistake was telling Roy that I just wanted to enjoy Thanksgiving through my Christmas birthday. I promised us that I'd head right back to the gym and martinet dieting once the holidays were over. I cut out pictures of fitness models from the dozen or so magazines I read each month and glued them to the resolution board above my work desk at home. Ever since my college days, I've been making a collage of my goals to keep reminding me of what I wanted to achieve that year. It's a bit silly, but it works—I've achieved every one of the goals I've ever set for myself. Except having the body I want.

Roy peeked over my shoulder at my little arts-and-crafts project.

"Is that the kind of body you want?" he said. I was sitting on the edge of the bed with the board on my lap, adding a picture of a woman with a solid six-pack and well-defined arms.

"Yeah. Do you think I can do it?"

"She's a fitness model; you need to remember that. This is what she does for a living." I was expecting him to say yes. This was not yes. This was the same guy who only months ago wasn't sure if my ass was a deal breaker, and now he was worried that I wanted to be too fit?

"I know, but if I work hard."

He stared at the picture. "I don't know if you have that body type . . . You would have to be very strict about your eating. And exercise like a demon."

I didn't know if there was much stricter that I could get with my eating. In my teen years there'd been a few times when I'd kept my calories under five hundred, but I was a grown-up. I couldn't function and work and think on fewer than eight hundred calories a day. Even that wasn't really sustainable.

"I am strict."

"I know, you look amazing," he said. I think sincerely, but I still took it as lip service. "I just don't want you to set yourself up for disappointment. I can tell you that that woman has a naturally thin body type. Putting muscle on is probably her biggest challenge. You have very different builds."

"I can do it," I told him, ending the discussion.

I was smaller than I've ever been—I was never a size six as an adult; even in my thin periods I was always an eight—and now that I knew I could get that small, I just wanted to keep getting smaller. It made me feel like I could do anything. I could have a body like a fitness model, and I could be an author. I wrote articles and blogs for a living, so I knew I could sell my words, but the longest thing I'd ever written was a twenty-three-page report on James Baldwin for my eleventh-grade English class. But now I had the confidence of a thinner person and decided to just send the bunch of personal essays I'd been working on to my agent.

She had taken me on as a client years earlier when I was working on a book proposal about how to make friends as an adult. Life got in the way and I never finished it, but she kept in touch and always asked me to send her whatever I was working on. I figured, *Why not? Just see where the world takes you.*

I wasn't sure I was ready to publish a book about my deepest, darkest secret—that I grew up with a father who's a hoarder—but writing about my childhood had been therapeutic. I spent my life trying to be perfect to compensate for how imperfect it used to be, and if I could write it all out, it might not have the power to hurt me anymore. And maybe sharing my story would help the cause, show people that hoarders aren't just a bunch of carny freaks to binge-watch on TV so you feel better about not doing the dishes. They're real people who hurt, people who have families who hurt.

I sent out the proposal and started taking meetings with publishers almost immediately. More often than not I heard that hoarding was passé. Like well-coiffed teenage vampires, my story had been around the block a few too many times. But in the end, two publishers made offers. I went with the one who promised to keep my family out of the press.

I had made a career out of confessing my insecurities to the world on the Internet, but this was different. I was petrified of what would happen when the book came out. There was a part of me, most of me really, that felt like once my secret was out, I would lose everything. My family would feel betrayed and stop loving me, my friends would be disgusted by me, and Roy would realize I wasn't quite as special as he thought I was. Writing the book was emotionally grueling, and I didn't have enough energy left to deal with anything else. I gave myself permission to do whatever I had to do to get through it, and eating topped the list. I ate without noticing. I ate to break up the monotony of long days spent in front of the computer. I ate to comfort myself as I cried for hours, forcing myself to dredge up every traumatic memory of my childhood. I ate when I remembered not having food at home for years because our kitchen had been abandoned to rats and maggots. I ate because I felt guilty and horrible, because by writing about my life I was hurting my family, and every word I typed was a stab in the back. I ate more than I had ever allowed myself to eat. I gained ten, then twenty, thirty, eventually forty pounds. It was as if all the weight that I'd ever kept at bay came back with a vengeance. I waited for Roy to break up with me, but he didn't. He told me he loved me and loved my body, whatever I weighed.

I didn't believe him. I knew he was lying. If I was too fat for him when we met, I must've been monstrous to him now. I did believe that he loved me: it was just that he did so despite my body. Two years passed between when we met and when I submitted *Coming Clean*, and in that time he hadn't missed a day of sending me a text to tell me he was thinking of me; he called regularly before we moved in together; and he never let two days pass without planning a night for us. He kept being wonderful, and I was just getting fatter and sadder and fatter.

One of the first things I did after sending in the manuscript was sign up for a half marathon as a means of getting back in shape. It was a charity race, so I was accountable to the training team and to the friends and family who sponsored me. It's easier to do things for other people. Every Saturday morning when I laced up for practice, I reminded myself that I was helping save kids with cancer—and that if I didn't run, I was an asshole who was killing kids with cancer. It was hard; I was heavier than I'd ever been and my knees hurt when I ran and the weight didn't come off like I wanted it to, but I kept at it, and I was proud of my progress.

On a Saturday morning after my long run, three months into my regimen, I broke my foot. I wasn't even running; I was texting with a friend whose husband had gained a lot of weight, giving her advice (I'm aware of the irony), when I tripped down the stairs of my third-floor walk-up.

My downstairs neighbor was walking into the building just as I was taking off my shoe—as if looking at my foot would tell me something—and offered to help me back up the stairs.

"No, I'm okay." I said. I wasn't okay. I knew it was broken right away. But I didn't want to have to put my weight on him. I didn't want him to feel how heavy I was. That was my only thought, sitting there with three flights of stairs to climb and a foot searing with pain.

I hobbled upstairs and called Roy, who rushed back home from the gym. He tried to carry me piggyback down the stairs and to the emergency clinic at the end of our street, but I was reluctant to put all my weight on him, so he hailed a cab to take us the two-and-a-half blocks.

It was a bad break—an avulsion fracture of my navicular bone—and it didn't heal right at first. It took months before I could walk without pain. Instead of running off my memoir weight, I was stuck on the couch, back to eating to pass the time until I could walk again. I gained back what I'd lost and then some.

I was emotionally and physically drained once again. Roy decided to book us a trip to Israel to celebrate the publishing of *Coming Clean* (and my newly regained perambulation). It wasn't the best move on our part: it was right in the middle of the press cycle, but I didn't care. I didn't think anyone was going to read it anyway, and I needed to get away from the book and the city and the tidal wave of emotion I'd been living in. Most of all, I needed to get away from GrubHub.

I'd been to Israel twice before. I'd already prayed at the Western Wall, floated in the Dead Sea, and climbed Masada; I told Roy I wanted to skip the tourist attractions and do something authentically Israeli when we got there.

"Eat hummus?" Roy said in his thickest Israeli accent. "Move furniture?"

"Something different," I told him.

"Okay, leave it to me."

Zimmer means "room" in German, but the Israelis have taken the word on as a synonym for "love shack," and the north of Israel is a hotbed of little romantic getaways. Before we left Roy had spent days upon days on Israeli Yelp-style sites looking at zimmers in the Golan Heights, each with its own romantic flavor: some boasted mood lighting and neon hot tubs, some had distressed wood and sheer white curtains photographed swaying in the mountain breeze, some looked like five-star hotel suites, some looked like Motel 6. He ended up choosing an idyllic wooden mountaintop cabin, far away from city lights. It took three busses and a hitchhike to get there, but when we finally arrived, we were treated to the breathtaking view of the Sea of Galilee sprawled beneath us.

The skies were clear, the air was fresh, and the atmosphere was completely serene—the exact opposite of New York City and exactly what I needed. Our cabin was furnished with an indoor hot tub and an outdoor pool-cuzzi (an enormous Jacuzzi or a very small pool; it was up for debate), a giant bed, and a variety of lounge chairs looking over the side of the mountain. A basket of wine, chocolates, and fruit waited for us on the counter. It was perfectly romantic and totally wasted on my exhausted mind and body. The combination of flights and bus rides and the last twelve months had worn me out, and when I walked in the door, I just continued walking to the bed and fell asleep.

When I woke up eight hours later, the sun was going down, bathing the surrounding mountains in a spectrum of orange and red, reflecting off the sea in blinding golden shimmers. It was paradise. Roy had arranged the dining table on the patio with dinner he'd had delivered.

Between bites I took pictures of the sunset and deep breaths of unpolluted air. As a kid I hated the quiet of the suburbs; I could never understand why my parents chose to leave the city for Long Island. But up on the mountain with nothing but the birds, I got it. Maybe you have to truly be tired to fully appreciate silence.

Roy looked calm and happy. He'd needed this vacation too. I wasn't the easiest person to live with over the past year. There had been a lot of crying, a lot of anger I directed at him unfairly, either because I was dealing with feelings I hadn't given myself room for before or just because I was stressing over a deadline. I was a bit of a sobbing, irascible mess. He never flinched; he took it all and promised me that I'd come out of this experience stronger. It was nice to see him relaxed. At home.

He took the opportunity to say a bunch of really nice things, which isn't a rarity for Roy. He's definitely the romantic one in our relationship, and usually I roll my eyes at my personal nineteenth-century poet, but I let it slide this time. For once it was an appropriate venue for such pontifications.

"Every day I'm with you," he told me, "I'm a better man for it. And if you'll let me, I'd like to spend every day of the rest of my life making you happy."

He leaned in to kiss me, and when I opened my eyes he was down on one knee.

"Kimberly Rae Miller, will you marry me?"

At this point I think he pulled out a ring, but I don't actually know, because I covered my face with my hands and refused to look at him.

"Shut up!" was the only thing I could say.

Totally overwhelmed. I should have known something was up, but I was so wrapped up in deadlines and rewrites that Roy could have been walking around in a diaper and speaking Swedish and I wouldn't have noticed.

I peeked from between my fingers, saw him and the ring, then said, "Shut up!" again.

To his credit, he laughed and waited patiently for me to stop crying and look at him, which I didn't, but I did eventually nod my head.

"Is that a yes?"

I couldn't really speak with all the crying, but I managed to say, "Yes."

He gently pried my hands away from my face so he could kiss me and put a ring on my finger. A ring he designed himself. Rose gold, with a braided band. It looked like the kind of ring you'd find in a museum, something from another time. Completely original, just like him.

I was in starry-eyed bliss for about five minutes before I started tallying the calories in the zimmer fridge. I needed to go on a wedding diet.

THREE

BROKEN BODIES

There's a magic number in weight loss: 1,200. That's how many calories it is simultaneously recommended a (female) dieter eat and not go below because they might end up in something called starvation mode. It has been dieting's golden rule since the days of Lulu Hunt Peters and her 1918 calorie counting manual *Diet and Health: With Key to the Calories.*

I must have written a dozen or so pieces over the course of my career that make reference to "not going below 1,200 calories" or a "healthy diet of 1,200 calories a day." It's so ubiquitous a standard that it doesn't even need citing, which is good because it's not actually based on any real science. There's never been a study that found that the human body loses weight optimally at a diet of 1,200 calories, nor one that proves the body's metabolic system is somehow adversely affected by a diet below 1,200 calories. The number of calories a person should eat to lose weight or can limit themselves to without having an adverse effect on their body's functioning varies from person to person, body to body, lifestyle to lifestyle; the only way to know your metabolic sweet spot for sure is to get your basal metabolic rate (BMR) tested. The 1,200-calorie rule is based on a formula for one woman: the average-in-every-way woman. It assumes that an average woman of average height and average age and average weight and average daily physical activity burns 2,100 calories per day. Basically, a woman of medium build who is between the ages of twenty-three and fifty, five foot four inches tall, around 130 pounds, who takes regular walks but is neither a gym rat nor couch potato, and who is in good physical health. It then uses the recommendation (by the American College of Sports Medicine)[1] that people lose no more than two pounds per week,[2] which requires a deficit of approximately seven thousand calories a week, therefore reducing one thousand calories a day and then rounding up by one hundred calories as a safety measure. In reality, 1,200 calories may be too much food for some people to successfully lose weight, especially those of a small build or a sedentary lifestyle, while it can be dangerously low for others.

I knew all of that when I decided that 1,200 calories was my number. I also knew all of that when I decided that one thousand calories was my number, and nine hundred calories was my number, and eight hundred calories was my number in all my previous years of dieting. I knew, or thought I knew, everything there was to know about dieting.

I knew the science of it, I knew the benefits and dangers of it, and I knew how to make it happen for my own body; dieting was the thing my world revolved around. While it used to be something I was ashamed of, the need to always be on a diet, the fact that I was marrying a personal trainer and had landed a job at a media company editing diet books and writing health blogs all day meant that I could be openly obsessed with dieting in a way that I never could before. Counting calories was no longer a dirty little secret (*hey, I'm not thin naturally; I have to deprive myself constantly—which is surprisingly something I do*

---

1.   Dr. Peters came up with the number based on her personal dietary habits. She was not the average-in-every-way-woman. She stood five foot seven inches, and her weight vacillated between 150 pounds and 230 pounds. The American College of Sports Medicine was not founded until 1954.

2.   This recommendation is based on research; for the general population, weight loss that exceeds two pounds per week may have a deleterious effect on bone and muscle mass.

not actually enjoy) but something one does as a diet industry insider, an expert. Which is why the weight gain I'd had while eating my way through my memoir made me so much more self-conscious than I'd ever been. I knew better. I had no excuse. I'd been so close to being the version of myself that I wanted to be, and I gave it all up because writing a book made me sad. I felt pathetic. And I had to fix it because I was getting married.

And so I chose 1,200 again because that was the number that *everyone* said I should aim for and because I wanted to do it all perfectly this time (and also because it was as low as the calorie-counting app on my phone would go). I had the relationship and the job, so now I was going to have a perfect life and a perfect weight loss. I would do it all by the book, nothing extreme.

I hired a personal trainer near my office so I wouldn't have an excuse to miss the gym, and woke up at five a.m. so I could get to the gym before the treadmills filled up with the prework crowd. I cooked all my meals over the weekend, weighing and measuring them out into homemade Lean Cuisines, and in the evenings after work I walked the three-and-a-half miles home. I did every single thing I had ever suggested others do, and I waited for the scale to move.

And it did.

It moved up.

163.

163.4.

165.

I couldn't stop gaining weight.

I sent daily food journals to my trainer-trainer and my fiancé-trainer, and when they were both incredulous about my calories, I started sending pictures of everything I ate to assure them my portions weren't enormous. They thought I was faking it, that I was eating things I wasn't supposed to, and I didn't blame them; I would have thought the exact same thing.

Roy asked his friend Yair Lahav, the director of both nutrition and strength-training studies at the Wingate Institute in Israel, where Roy had gone to school and worked, to put together a clinical diet for me, the kind of diet they use in hospitals to check for hormone issues. For a week I ate diet bread (which has an unfathomable amount of unhealthy ingredients) and cans of tuna and egg whites and vegetables. I didn't lose an ounce.

I went to my doctor for a physical and got my yearly thyroid check and prayed that that was it; I could just take a pill and be back on my calorie-restricting way. My mother had Hashimoto's disease, an autoimmune disease where your immune system attacks your thyroid. She'd found out about it when I was in high school, and because it's often passed down from the maternal line, I was immediately tested. The tests came back positive for the antibodies; my thyroid hormone levels were always low, but not so low that my doctor felt the need to medicate them. "You just need to exercise a little more than other people," my general practitioner had told me. And I did. And it worked. Nothing had changed in the last fifteen years: my tests came back positive for Hashimoto's antibodies and slightly lower thyroxin levels than were ideal, but nothing to worry about.

I had dieted successfully on a slightly screwed-up thyroid most of my life. Now nothing was working. I was supposed to be my most beautiful self on my wedding day, but I had reached a point where I refused to even look in a mirror or go out in public. I declined the engagement party my parents wanted to throw us, not wanting there to be any photographic evidence of my existence, and I started to feign feeling tired or sick whenever Roy planned a date night that involved other people.

"People are starting to think we broke up, Kim." He very rarely got angry with me. My social awkwardness was the price he paid for falling in love with an introvert, but he was mad at me. I'd crossed a line when

I'd started encouraging him to go out to events alone—a compromise, I thought—so he could still be social and I could still be invisible.

"At least let me post a picture of us together on Facebook," he pleaded.

"I'm sorry," I said, and I meant it. "Not right now."

"Our wedding album is just going to be pictures of me, isn't it?"

I didn't say anything, but I wished it could be. He looked great.

"I'm trying. I just can't lose weight this time. I don't know what's wrong."

"I don't know either," he said. My weight had become a constant topic of conversation. As we sat down for dinner I'd go over my food journal with him, showing him pictures of my meals throughout the day so he could assess portion sizes and nutrient makeup. He was the trainer and I was the client, and every once in a while when he could distract me enough so that I'd forget to hate myself, I would also be his fiancée.

"I don't know how to help you anymore, babe," he said. "I feel helpless."

"I'm sorry I'm like this," I said. "I fuck everything up."

"I think that's a little hyperbolic," he said, trying to make me laugh away the tears that were obviously verging. "Your body is tricky. That's all. Maybe you should see a nutritionist."

"They're expensive," I told him. Our wedding was already an enormous financial drain on our lives; I didn't want my body to be too.

"I'll pay anything to see you happy again," he said. "And I'd like it if you'd go outside once in a while."

I'd found the nutrition practice on a list of New York's best doctors. The founding partner was the nutrition consultant for a morning show. I couldn't afford to see her. The cheapest nutritionist they had was $225 an hour, and so that's who I booked my appointment with, hoping that spending a small fortune would ensure that I was clued in to some magic dietary secret that only those with an RD degree, and the people who paid them, were privy to.

I'd used the bathroom three times between leaving my office and stopping in a Starbucks, a shoe store, and the building's lobby before finally ringing the bell. I used to do that on the way to Weight Watchers meetings in hopes I could drain every ounce of excess liquid from my system before getting on a scale in front of a stranger.

I'd picked the latest possible appointment because my work schedule was always a little unpredictable. The nutritionist's office was already dimmed; the secretaries had already gone home for the day and turned the decorative lamps placed around the waiting room off, leaving only the faint fluorescent ones in their place. Three of the four offices were empty and dark, but I could hear voices behind the one closed door.

I'd had actual nightmares about this appointment, something akin to showing up naked to school, only this time I was in my frumpiest underwear on a scale in front of the whole building that just happened to be made up of everyone I knew. I knew it was silly; I was paying this woman to be nice to me, but that didn't mean I wasn't apprehensive about the lecture on calories and vegetables I was sure I was going to get, and how defensive I would sound when I told her that I knew how to diet, I just didn't know why it didn't work anymore. I was compiling a little speech in my head of books I'd edited and the fitness certifications I had under my belt if she questioned my inherent knowledge of calories and fitness. I made my own almond milk and baked my own bread from wheat berries I ground into flour in a blender that cost more than my first car; we kept a vegetarian home and made most things from scratch. The only processed food in our house came in the form of protein powder.

She wouldn't believe me. I wouldn't have believed me.

As I heard the women behind the door start to exchange good-byes, I prepared myself for the inevitable, trying to look friendly and approachable, sitting up straight and tucking my hair behind my ears.

When the door opened, two young women walked out. Girls, I thought, they looked like girls. I'd expected the nutritionist who greeted me at the door to be a wiry middle-aged woman, with frizzy hair and a no-nonsense demeanor, preferably wearing Eileen Fisher—actually, I imagined Annie Potts would be my nutritionist. Or Mary Steenburgen, I would settle for Mary Steenburgen.

Instead, Alison was a bubbly twenty-six-year-old with a Long Island accent (takes one to know one). I thought she was the intern, but she assured me she had graduated from her Ivy League nutrition program and was a fully certified member of the professional staff.

She had an eagerness that made me nervous but was also sort of endearing—I remembered being fresh from school and wanting so desperately for people to take me seriously, and for the most part people had given me the benefit of the doubt. Alison wore a combination of blazer and maxi dress in what I assume was an attempt to look professional before she'd saved enough money to invest in a work wardrobe.

Who was I to judge? I refused to buy new clothes. My closet was still full of size sixes and eights that I hadn't worn in years. Instead I wore the same pair of fat pants with one of many cardigans every single day. Cardigans are like the security blankets of clothes, hiding muffin tops and covering straining fabric seams. Or at least that's what I told myself.

Alison assured me that I wasn't the first person to come in after years of dieting unable to lose the weight I'd gained. I remained skeptical; she couldn't possibly be experienced enough to have met a lot of people like me. But I supposed that everyone who came in here said that they were doing everything right.

I'd filled out a questionnaire before our meeting, carefully detailing my history of dieting from skipping lunch in elementary school to the seven-hundred- to eight-hundred-calorie days I'd decreased to when I met Roy. The questionnaire also covered my food preferences and allergies (blueberries) and what my goals were. She was more concerned

with my emotional history and my need to diet excessively since childhood than she was about my upcoming wedding. I already had a therapist, and I was reluctant to trust that my newly minted dietician could
handle the breadth of my emotional baggage. I considered bringing
her a copy of my memoir *Coming Clean* and saying, "All my issues are
in here." Except that I didn't believe in blaming my own shortcomings
on my family. My father's hoarding had certainly shaped the person I
became, but I wanted to believe that it shaped me for the better, had
made me stronger and harder working, not someone who was as obsessive about food and dieting as he was about stuff.

Instead I told Alison about my childhood as a child actor and
dancer, how there had always been a lot of pressure on me to be thin,
and that no matter how much I tried I never seemed to get thin enough
for anyone's liking. It was cliché and easy to understand, and it worked.
My past was my past; I was more concerned with the future. The immediate future—my wedding was four months away.

She listened attentively and took notes, nodding when appropriate,
all while reviewing months of my carefully recorded entries in my online
food journal, my recent blood work and thyroid panel, and the results
of a BMR test I'd taken the week before our meeting. After scrutinizing
everything about me that I was so incredibly insecure about, my svelte
former-figure-skater nutritionist gave me some bad news: my body had
no idea what to do with food anymore. Years of eating below my most
basic caloric needs coupled with significant exercise had left my body
perfectly conditioned to survive during the 1930s dust bowl without a
problem, but in the chia seed–smoothie, Whole Foods, Upper West
Side life I was living, I couldn't eat a modest diet of 1,200 calories a
day. For my superefficient metabolism, this was considered overeating.
"Eat less, move more" was a mantra I had lived by, but I'd taken it to
extremes for more than half my life, and I had broken my body.

"Your resting metabolic rate is less than nine hundred calories. I can't encourage you to eat less than that. We need to build your metabolism back up," she said.

"Great!" I said, always overly enthusiastic when I'm nervous. "How do we do that?"

Alison explained that I needed to eat more—and carefully. By eating healthy foods—foods I already eat—I'd have to increase my calories slowly.

I could feel some tears forming.

"I'm going to be huge for my wedding," I said, mostly to myself.

"You're going to be beautiful on your wedding day, no matter what you weigh. You need to do this." She sounded like a combination of my fiancé and my mother—it was condescending. I didn't want to be coddled. I wanted to be thin.

At the end, it was decided that eventually my goal was to get up to 1,800 calories a day, which was about right for someone my size (fourteen) and activity level (minimal during my memoir-writing stage, about an hour a day of real physical activity now).

"But we'll increase slowly," Alison assured me.

I had never in my life allowed myself to eat up to 1,800 calories unless I was binging.

Eating slowly to allow my body to eventually adjust to 1,800 calories and . . . no cardio. Alison said that my body needed to start getting used to *using* calories and not just storing them for survival.

After hearing this, I wanted to run out of her office and hide in the abandoned subway tunnels with the Mole People. If I were a normal person, Alison's "eat more, move less" plan would have sounded amazing. I'd always dreamed of a day when I wouldn't have to exercise so hard, when I didn't have to track every calorie burned on my heart-rate monitor to ensure I'd done enough to justify eating, but not now. Not four months before my wedding. Of all the diets she could have asked of me, this was the worst.

Eighteen hundred calories; double what I was currently burning efficiently.

In 1944, as World War II was coming to a close, thirty-six men volunteered for what would become the most famous study about the physical and psychological effects of starvation: the Minnesota Starvation Study, run by Ancel Keys at the University of Minnesota.

Europe was faced with hordes of starved victims of the war and needed to know what they were dealing with and how to feed these survivors back to health. The men in the study started off eating a healthy 3,200 calories a day, the amount required to maintain their weight. They were eventually reduced to 1,800 calories a day, coupled with twenty-two miles of required walking a week. By the end of the six-month experiment, the men reported feelings of severe emotional distress, depression, and anxiety, distraction and an inability to think clearly, and obsessive thoughts about food. One man cut off a few fingers with an axe and couldn't remember why.

When the study ended the participants were allowed to "refeed." Keys's team observed the participants under two separate stages: in the first they were allotted more food, but in controlled quantities; in the second they were allowed to eat until they felt sated. The latter group ate up to ten thousand calories a day. The weight they'd lost came back at an astounding rate. At the end of the twenty-week recovery period, they had an average increase in body fat of 50 percent, in what researchers would dub "poststarvation obesity." While many were still at a normal body weight, their muscle mass had decreased significantly while their fat mass had increased significantly and their basal metabolic rates had dropped.

I had first heard of the Minnesota Starvation Study years earlier while reading Gina Kolata's *Rethinking Thin* and subsequently devoured everything I could find about it. The story struck a chord with me, but not as a cautionary tale; I wanted to know how far I could push my body. I smugly thought, *That's still a lot of food.* In my own perverse way, I was proud of my ability to eat so much less and put in so much more physical effort than a mere twenty-two miles a week of walking.

I thought about the men of that study as I sat across from Alison, whom I saw as giving me a dietary death sentence. I thought about all the diets I wrote about, all the diets I'd been on. I was stuck in an endless loop of starving and refeeding.

The whole process went against my diet writer/editor grain, but what had worked for the last twenty-four years of my dieting history was no longer working, so it was worth a shot.

Alison asked me to read a book about intuitive eating before our next meeting because she hoped it would help me understand our ultimate goal. I downloaded it to my tablet before even leaving the building, a little light reading for the train ride home. What became immediately obvious to me as I delved into my homework was that I had no idea what eating intuitively meant. It had been years since I felt hungry; I didn't remember what those pangs felt like. I could probably go days without eating and never feel that twinge of hunger the book suggested I look out for. I'd spent years alternating between eating on a schedule that was supposed to keep my metabolism burning efficiently and eating with wild abandon, rebelling against my self-imposed structure. Hunger was never an option, and I had no concept of being sated—either I ate until my carefully portioned meals were finished or I ate until I hated myself.

When I got home from my first appointment with Alison, Roy was waiting for me. He liked to sit down with me after my weekly therapy session to see if I'd had any emotional epiphanies I wanted to share or things that I wanted him to be more sensitive about. I guess starting our relationship off with a memoir meant that he felt really invested in my mental health, so he liked to have regular check-ins about what I was feeling. It was a little like living with a sexy Dr. Phil: thoughtful, a little intrusive, well meaning, and sometimes helpful. In a similar posttherapy check-in fashion, I told him about my metabolism-fixing meal plan. I could see his trainer face twisting into skepticism, and I assured him that this was not carte blanche to eat whatever I want but a careful combination of healthy foods that I already ate and in tiered caloric increases.

As I retold Roy everything Alison planned for me, I could feel myself already dreading what was ahead. The plan felt daunting. The book I'd just started reading had said that I needed to break away from my constant obsessing about food, but my tiered meal plan required diligent attention to what I ate.

I told him that in layperson's terms I had damaged my metabolism after years of eating too little. He was doubtful, but said it was worth a try.

"I don't know," he said. "Your metabolism isn't an organ; you can't break it. It's the rate between building and destroying tissue, and an intricate combination of systems: hormonal, thermoregulatory, biome-chanical . . . There are no instances of people leaving periods of extreme caloric deprivation heavier."

And yes, he does actually speak like that.

I was frustrated, and the science Roy detailed wasn't working for me. This seemed like my only solution.

"Give it a try," he said. "I may be reticent to completely agree with this prognosis, but I will admit that you have one of the most obstinate bodies I've ever dealt with in my career."

An obstinate body—now that was marriage material.

Earlier, while reading about intuitive eating on the subway ride home, I'd had the sort of emotional epiphany one has on public trans-portation while attempting to undertake a dietary life change: I needed to tell Roy about reading his email about me years earlier. I had carried his words with me every day of our lives together. Not the good ones, not the ones where he wrote that I was *pretty much perfect*. I focused on being "chunky" and that my big butt and belly really bothered him. He had never said anything to me about my weight, not in the three years we'd been together, but he was always very eager to help me lose weight when I talked about being unhappy with myself—and I took his support as proof enough that he wasn't attracted to me. And I resented him for it. Love is something that's supposed to be unconditional, but I felt like I had to earn his through starvation. Maybe I wasn't trying hard enough; maybe I was gaining weight to test him. Maybe I was a lot more screwed up than I thought.

I hadn't told Alison about his email, how it had held a prime spot at the forefront of my mind all the time, another motivator in my losing weight, but I felt like I needed to come clean to Roy. I needed to lay it all out there if this was going to work, if I was really going to fix my relationship with myself.

He was done with our check-in, but I wasn't. I followed him into our bedroom where he was changing into pj's.

"I need to tell you something. Something I did—you're going to be mad at me," I told Roy after some hesitation.

I sat down on our bed and looked up at him. This was a mistake. Our life was good. We were happy. We were getting married, and I was about to confess to doing something really uncool.

"What did you do?" The color drained from his face. I could see he was thinking the worst: I cheated on him, or I ruined his *Avengers #4* from 1963, his most prized possession.

I assured him it wasn't *that* bad. Okay, it was bad—I had invaded his privacy a long time ago—but it's not what Roy was thinking of as "bad."

I was petrified he would never talk to me again for having betrayed his trust.

"Do you regret it?" he asked.

I told him I did, and he waved it off and said I didn't have to confess.

Which was tempting, but I had to—not to clear my conscience but because it had been eating away at me for almost our entire relationship.

"When we first started dating, I didn't trust you. I thought you were a player." He slowly shook his head—that much he already knew. "I thought I was just some placeholder for when a hotter girl came around, so I read your email one night while you were at work."

He was still standing above me, looking down. He didn't look mad. He looked amused and a little confused, like, *Why would you want to do that?*

"You had written to Geoff about me. You said that you liked me a lot, but that I was fat—and you weren't sure if that was a deal breaker."

His face sank, and I waited for him to yell at me, but he didn't.

"I'm so sorry. I was a different guy then," he said. He looked ashamed. Not the reaction I was expecting. "My priorities were screwed up."

"You're not mad that I read your email?" I asked, since that was really the only thing I could wrap my head around at the moment.

"I'm certainly not thrilled about it, but I'm not mad at you—I'm mad at me for writing something so hurtful. I was living in a different world then. A superficial world. If it makes you feel better, I got over it really quickly. Your weight became a nonissue for me."

I didn't believe him. He gave me no reason not to, but I didn't.

"You could gain fifty pounds and I wouldn't care, Kim."

"I *have* gained fifty pounds."

"And I proposed to you. And I'm marrying you. I don't care about your weight. I care about you . . . I'm sorry I was an asshole." He came over and wrapped his arms around me.

"You were an asshole in private, to be fair."

"Why didn't you tell me this then?"

"Because we were new, and I was being crazy, and you would have broken up with me."

"Why didn't you break up with me?"

"I thought about it. But I liked you."

"I'm glad you didn't," he said. "I'm sorry."

"Me too."

———

It took about two months and $2,000 in nutritionist bills to stop gaining weight. "Fixing" my metabolism was a slower process than I cared for. Once I went a few weeks without gaining a pound, Alison increased my food allotment. And once my weight plateaued I was allotted a second yogurt a day or a palm full of nuts and so on and so on. She wouldn't let me track my calories, but instead worked out meal plans that only she could see the nutrient breakdown of. But I'd been counting calories since elementary school—I kept a mental tally and tried to keep my anxiety in check with each one-hundred-calorie increase. On my wedding day I was up to 1,700 calories and had lost three pounds. Three whole pounds.

I didn't feel beautiful the day I got married. It was a beautiful day. Everything was perfect, but I felt wrong.

Roy looked amazing. He was wearing a Brioni tuxedo, the same one that Daniel Craig wore in *Casino Royale*.

I wore a dress. A very simple A-line dress with a sweetheart neckline: there was no bling or flourish, just a simple white dress. It was classic and it flattered me. No matter my size, my hips and waist have always had a ten-inch difference, and the dress accentuated my proportions.

I was happy that I even found a dress I liked. I hated the entire wedding-dress-shopping process. I hated having to look at myself in mirrors for hours in dresses that were too small for me, trying to imagine what they would look like if they were the right size. I went to the dress shop alone—I didn't really want anyone else's opinion on what I should wear on my wedding day, and I didn't want anyone to gush over me and tell me how beautiful I was. I just wanted to get it over with. The dresses I liked online and in bridal magazines were lacey and delicate, but all the lace dresses I'd tried on accentuated the roundness of my abdomen and hips and the enormity of my breasts that had gone from a C cup to double D. So I chose a simple, flattering A-line dress the designer assured me was the right dress for me.

My mother was hurt.

"A wedding is something a girl and her mother do together," she told me. There were some logical fallacies in her statement, but I'd hurt her and apologized—for months. I'd screwed up yet again. But being a fat bride was not something I wanted to revel in. I didn't want to see my mother tear up at beautiful dresses or tell salespeople what a beautiful little girl I had been or how she had always dreamed of this day for me. I wasn't even sure I wanted a real wedding with all the attention on me. A city-hall wedding, a cardigan, and a selfie might be enough for me.

"You'll regret it later if you don't. I did," my mother told me when I championed the benefits of a city-hall marriage. My parents married four days after I was born in the office of a Methodist church after work one evening. My mother is Jewish, my father Catholic; they figured Methodist was a compromise. I could compromise too; I could have a traditional wedding without letting myself feel like a bride.

I planned our wedding like I was planning a birthday party: party dress, favors, cake, invitations, check, check, check. I didn't want to get too invested. I didn't like being the center of attention. And I was able to keep up that "who cares, it's just my wedding" act until the exact moment my maid of honor, Anna, zipped up my wedding dress in the bridal suite and I started sobbing uncontrollably.

"I was wondering when this would happen," she said. "You've been way too calm."

I wasn't nervous about getting married; I was nervous about everyone looking at me, at everyone remembering me on this day looking like this. And I just wanted to be with Roy—he would help me keep all my anxiety in check. Roy loved parties; I loved sitting at home in sweatpants. I'd never done well in big social gatherings, and Roy had always hammed things up and taken the attention on himself when I needed to fade into the background. He couldn't do that for me today—people like brides; they like talking to them and taking pictures with them and telling them how beautiful they look.

I couldn't stop crying, and the photographer looked at me like I was nuts. She needed to do the bridal portrait, she told me, as if that were somehow reason enough to get my shit together. I didn't want a portrait. I wanted to go find Roy.

He was waiting on a pier with his back to me. It was all so silly, so fake: a setup for pictures that were supposed to be romantic. Every day of our life was so much more naturally romantic than this. I was tempted to push him, to jump in the water after him. To do something that would make this whole thing less contrived.

He was silent when he turned around, and then he touched my face with his thumb to wipe away a tear. And then he started tearing up.

"This is exactly what I thought you'd look like," he said.

I'd never really appreciated how beautiful Long Island was when I was growing up. I'd never given much thought to the ubiquitous beaches, clear skies, and salt-imbued air that engulfed the tiny strip of land. Everything beautiful about my hometown was in full display on the day Roy and I got married. We'd found a venue a few minutes from where I'd grown up, on the Great South Bay, and I allowed the fact that I was home to comfort me in a way it never had before. The dress and makeup and formality of the day were completely outside my comfort zone, but the cool bay air and squawking of seagulls were soothing in a way that only home can be.

The ferry to Fire Island left from a port just a hundred yards from where we were standing, and the ferry captain tooted his horn and the passengers screamed their congratulations and waved at us, breaking the spell of the moment and ushering us on to our next call of duty: getting married.

I'd asked a dear friend who had grown up to be a legal mastermind but had toured the festival circuit as part of a ska band in his youth to dust off his trumpet for the occasion. The first few notes of "Just the Way You Are" were our cue that it was time to take our places.

Walking down the aisle was the best part of the day. Roy looked happier than I'd ever seen him. My closest friends and all my family smiling, I decided to just let myself enjoy this day. Even if I wasn't what I thought was my ideal, beautiful self, I gave myself this one day to be happy.

———

I kept up my reverse diet even after the wedding, but I stopped paying to see Alison. Roy and I wanted to buy an apartment or a house and have kids, and I needed that money to go toward the things that really mattered. Maintaining my overweight status just didn't feel all that important.

My reverse-dieting plan was just as strict as any of the deprivation diets I'd been on. My life still revolved around food—I was just eating more of it. Spending my days obsessing over eating enough calories to keep my metabolism functioning felt just as disordered as spending my days obsessing over restricting my calories for optimal weight loss. Now that I was burning calories again, I didn't know what to do to reduce them without screwing my system up again. I wanted a life that didn't involve obsessing over everything I ate, but how would I get to that point?

I was burnt out on obsessing. I was going to have to come to terms with the facts that a) I may never get back to my ideal weight, and b) my ideal weight might not be ideal in regard to the amount of effort needed to maintain it as a working, socially active, soonish-to-be-child-bearing member of society. I would have to take the advice I'd been dispensing to blog readers for years: I would have to find a way to eat well and be okay with my body as it is, as it maybe, just maybe, was meant to be.

I had spent the majority of my life trying to fit a mold that didn't work for my body—and it fought me tooth and nail. I didn't know what my ideal body would look like. "Somebody else's" came to mind, but that wasn't going to happen. I needed to find the body that wouldn't mean a life of starvation and a twenty-hour-a-week gym commitment, but that also wouldn't mean hiding from the world at large.

I knew my body's set point—a weight that was relatively easy for me to maintain with little effort. In the past it had been 145, but at five foot five inches, that was always a little heavier than I was comfortable with, and I was already so far from that point. Every time I had reached a goal weight in my past I had found a new flaw to focus on. I'd never let myself simply be thin enough.

I wanted to know what it was I was really supposed to look like, not based on the pictures in the magazines I worked for or the recommendations of the diet experts whose books I edited. I had spent a lifetime dieting, and it had made me heavier.

We seem to know everything about everything, but we still don't know why some of us have "good" metabolisms and "bad" metabolisms. We don't know why some people are short and stocky and some are long and lean. There had to be some reason, some biological reason.

I'd finally made some progress in regard to my BMR, so I didn't want to push my body to the extremes of my past. But I still needed to lose weight. To like looking at myself in the mirror again, to care what I wore and take pictures with my new husband without strategically hiding half my body behind him. Without a wedding, without a $6,000 diet-pill-model contract to win, without a child pageant to compete in, I was at a loss as to what I should strive for this time around. I didn't have a specific weight or calorie goal to hit, but my whole life had been about achieving the unachievable, especially considering the diktats of my build. I started to really think, why do I have this body? What can I do with it; what can it look like? What *should* I look like?

I needed better sources. I needed to go to the library.

EVOLVING
VENUSES

Hohle Fels Venus is fat. She has enormous breasts, a big round belly, and thick thighs, and she brandishes her large vulva proudly. She is approximately thirty-five thousand years old—predating agriculture—and was carved from mammoth ivory during the Upper Paleolithic era in what is now Germany. She is the oldest known sculpture of the human form, and while she doesn't have an actual BMI, one would describe her as obese.

Most of the "Venus figurines" of the Upper Paleolithic period (forty thousand to ten thousand years ago) share Hohle Fels's body type. Since the artists aren't available to interview, historians have come up with multiple theories about the prevalence of corpulence in this early human art. These Venuses could be realistic depictions of individual women, or represent an ideal standard of beauty, or serve as fertility symbols. They might be depictions of a long-since-forgotten goddess or serve as homages to ancestors. We don't really know. But even if the Venuses were exaggerations and not depictions of common human form, their realistic shape and proportionality tell us that people of the area were no strangers to body fat. And what we can gather from this is that humans have always been fat.

Not all of us, surely, but some of us have always been fat. Depictions of our cave-dwelling ancestors in textbooks and wax dioramas at natural history museums never seem to have an ounce of extra body fat, but our ancestors in the last glacial era were familiar with the way the body curves and stretches in the expanse of fat. Women with big hips, stomachs, and breasts were a regular-enough occurrence in that thirty-thousand-year gap to consistently be the subject of Upper Paleolithic carvings. There have been fat humans for as long as there have been humans. The current Paleo diet trend idealizes the nutrition of these long-dead people who had life expectancies that peaked in their thirties, as if they were pillars of natural health and instinctually knew better than to get fat. But the truth is that for most of human history, our ancestors simply had less food available and had to work much harder for it. Whether they got fat or not and when they did have access to food had more to do with where they lived than instinct and self-control.

I'd learned about evolution in seventh-grade Life Science class, and I was immediately obsessed with finding out what it meant for me: how I could change myself, how I could be better.

My obsession may have been partially fueled by my unrequited love for my science teacher, Mr. Cohen. He was a small man, maybe an inch or two taller than I was, probably in his midthirties—though years of teaching seemed to be prematurely graying him—but he was smart and funny, and my adolescent love for him was pure and true. He was married with children and not a pedophile, and so for all of these reasons he did not reciprocate my feelings, but that didn't deter my crush in the slightest. I internalized every word he said. His classes on cell structure and endoplasmic reticulum and mitochondria were brilliant, and maybe also contained veiled messages of his unbridled adoration for me. When he'd chuckled over the absurdity of old misconceptions like Aristotle's theory of spontaneous generation, I'd blush and chortle along with him. *Silly Aristotle, thinking that maggots sprang to life from dead flesh.*

The day Mr. Cohen introduced genetics and evolution to my twelve-year-old brain, my life was forever changed. According to Mr. Cohen, everything about us was predetermined at the moment we were conceived: our hair color, our eye color, our height, our build. Nature had been weeding out inferior genes for millennia via natural selection. We were the best of the best of the best millions of years of evolution had to offer.

So why did I feel so inferior? Genetics was a perfect excuse for all my many imperfections and a valid reasoning point for why my friends could eat cookies without feeling bad about themselves and I couldn't. Everything I didn't like about myself I could blame on my ~~dad~~ bad genes. It wasn't my fault I had big thighs and broad shoulders or that I couldn't tan. I took after a pale, thickset Germanic man. My family had played a cruel joke on me. It wasn't fair.

Why hadn't natural selection made me—made us all—skinny? After all, wouldn't the better, prettier, skinnier genes win over time, relegating the genes that made us fat to the garbage bin of evolution?

I had so many questions about DNA and evolution, questions that my textbook didn't answer, so I decided to make evolution my science-fair project. The science fair was the smart, quiet, overzealous student equivalent of homecoming—being chosen to represent your grade before the district was like being crowned queen of the awkward kids. Mr. Cohen was in charge of approving our projects before we embarked on decorating our project boards. My hypothesis was that human beings, along with dogs (because I couldn't understand how my cocker spaniel and my rottweiler could be classified as the same species), are unique to the animal kingdom in that, while we share a genus and species with the rest of our kind, we look vastly different from one another, taking on a variety of shapes.[1] It's not like there are fat horses or squat giraffes or thick-winged birds.

Mr. Cohen ended up shooting down my brilliant science project idea (which cost him my affection) on account of it being "too complicated to prove," but the nagging question of why evolution hadn't taken care of my thighs has always remained.

As a reasonable and reasonably educated adult, I understand the biology. Weight gain and loss is a simple equation: we gain weight because we take in more calories than our body needs to fuel its functioning. We lose weight by expending more energy than we take in as calories in our food. What isn't quite that simple is determining just how many calories each of us needs to achieve our personally, medically, or socially acceptable body—whatever our goal is. Our bodies don't come off an assembly line. Two people of similar weight, height, body shape, and lifestyle can eat the same foods but with vastly different results. Some people require fewer calories than others. Their bodies are models of metabolic efficiency: they seem to hardly need any food at all to function in the world, and if they were to eat the recommended amount of food suggested by governing guidelines, they would actually gain weight. Their body is a great betrayer, who can bump up the needle on the scale in one moderately indulgent weekend.

Then there are a lucky few who have metabolic cycles that essentially burn off excess fuel as it enters the body, regardless of their energy output, people with coveted "good metabolisms" who seem to maintain a slim build regardless of eating habits. Although to be fair, men and women of this type have a harder time building muscle for the same

---

1.   I wasn't completely wrong in my assumption as a seventh grader. A 2009 study by researchers at Queen's and McGill Universities in Canada compared levels of variation in height and body mass among ninety-nine human populations and 848 animal populations, and found that although humans show low levels of height variation, they do have a distinctively high within-population body-mass variation.

reason that they have a hard time retaining body fat. Most of us are somewhere in between these two, but most of us also feel firmly we're the former. I do.

Which is why I was at the library researching a tiny figurine of an obese Upper Paleolithic woman. I had recently been tasked at work with finding a newer, sexier take on the Paleo diet when I'd come across Ms. Fels.

What did real Paleo people eat? Anything they could. If she were real, Hohle Fels Venus would have spent the majority of her day in shelter, probably sedentary, hiding from the elements of Europe during the Ice Age. Eating was probably the most exciting part of her day. She wasn't all that different from a modern office worker. Which is probably why she was so overweight.

The simple fact that she was obese piqued my interest. Were there so many mammoth carcasses lying around to gorge on that people ate to excess,[2] or were some of them prone to obesity? And if so, why? There had to be a reason—a usefulness for bodies like mine—that I was missing. There has to be a reason for everyone's body. And I was convinced that the answer had to be at the library. It certainly wasn't on the Internet because according to the Internet, anyone could look like a Victoria's Secret model if they weren't such lazy, worthless slobs.[3] And so there I was, past Patience and Fortitude, holed up in an office in the New York Public Library.

---

2. The most modern woolly mammoth dinner was surprisingly recent; in January 1951 the forty-seventh annual Explorers Club Dinner, held at the Roosevelt Ballroom in New York City, boasted a menu with recently discovered and thawed 250,000-year-old woolly mammoth meat. The cost per plate was $475.94, a bargain.

3. I also had to wonder about our devolution in regards to socializing, thanks to technology. Would future generations be born hunched and pale, with no survival skills but a keen ability to insult others anonymously?

Richard the Librarian bobbed his head, humming, uncertain about what exactly I was looking for but willing to humor me. After I'd shot down his list of historical standards of beauty, we spent the rest of our meeting going over how to use the journal database: evolution is a pretty robust topic in the scientific community (go figure), and I had my work cut out for me. Sorting through books and journals about human evolution became a project that slowly took over all my free time and mental space. I should have been in newlywed bliss—Roy and I had been married for less than a month, and instead of cuddling with my brand-new husband at the end of the day, I'd sit next to him in bed with a book in hand and a pile by my side and say things like, "Did you know white people have only been around for eight thousand years?"[4]

"That's interesting," he said, stroking my hair and kissing my forehead, then cheek, then neck, a gallant but futile attempt at starting some foreplay. But I had evolution on the brain.

"How do you think skinheads would feel about that?" I asked.

"I don't think they're open for a rational debate about their feelings of superiority," he responded, continuing to plant little sensuous kisses, undeterred by me bringing up Nazis in my pillow talk.

I patted his head and fell back into my reading, a long article full of nomenclature about evolutionary adaptations during the last Ice Age. He eventually gave up, opting to watch some TV since it was easier to turn on.

I was beginning to think this whole flight of fancy was an enormous waste of my evenings and weekends. I wasn't finding what I was looking

---

4.   Light skin tones were an adaptation of the later Ice Age, probably brought about by a genetic mutation that proved beneficial for survival. Skins with less melanin, and therefore lighter skin tones, attract vitamin D, while those with more melanin and darker skin tones have a harder time synthesizing vitamin D from the sun, though they do have some natural defense against sun damage, which would be beneficial to living in areas of the world with higher sun exposure.

for, and I wasn't going to find it in publications about the changing hip widths in early hominids.[5]

At the bottom of a journal article defending the long-slighted intelligence and cultural contributions of our Neanderthal cousins—a random tangent I kept on reading out of interest—I saw the names Allen and Bergmann. Their respective findings, according to the notes section, could explain the short, broad, and muscular build of *Homo neanderthalensis*.

Roy and I had taken a popular mail-order genetic test about a year earlier just for fun, and I'd found out that I was more Neanderthal than most, with a whopping 2.8 percent Neanderthal DNA in my system (it ranges from 1 percent to 4 percent, with Europeans averaging 2.7 percent). It would've been nice to blame these genes inherited from long-extinct ancestors for my build, but I quickly found out that most researchers believe that Neanderthal DNA in our *Homo sapiens* gene pool has little to no impact on our current species.

Still, this was the first lead I had, and I wanted to see if it was anything meaningful. Turns out, Allen and Bergmann and their biological rules are widely accepted among the evolutionary-science crowd.

Carl Bergmann was an early nineteenth-century German anatomist, physiologist, and biologist who in 1847 identified a pattern that would come to be known as Bergmann's Rule. His theory was pretty simple: the body mass of an animal—say, a human—is in direct relationship to the climate in which it lives. This means that animals found in cold climates tend to have greater body mass in smaller bodies, allowing them to produce more body heat. The opposite can be seen in animals living in warmer climates: larger surface areas in relation to body mass allows them to dissipate heat quickly and cool off the body efficiently.

---

5. Though it's worth noting that in our early hominid (mid-chimp-to-human) version, our hips were much wider than they are now, making childbirth a whole lot easier but upright walking significantly harder.

Joseph Allen was a late nineteenth-century zoologist, biologist, and curator at the American Museum of Natural History. In 1877, thirty years after Bergmann, he observed that animals in the same species (particularly endotherms, or warm-blooded species) varied in size and stature based on their geographical location. Mammals in high and low global latitudes, which have cold climates, have stockier trunks and shorter limbs, while mammals of the same species evolved in warm climates have leaner frames and longer limbs.

Like Bergmann, he also hypothesized that it was a result of the need to conserve or expend warmth; in cold climates, shorter limbs mean less heat escapes vital organs, and in warm climates longer limbs provide more surface area to disperse and dissipate heat.[6]

Because these two rules are complementary, they tend to be mentioned in unison, and together they explain this: human beings whose ancestors lived in cold climates are inclined to have stocky frames, with short limbs and more muscle and fat mass, all of which are advantageous to maintaining body heat in times of harsh temperatures. Alternatively, people whose ancestors hail from hot climate regions tend to have longer limbs and lither bodies, best suited to cooling off quickly.

Short legs. Broad build. Ability to retain fat and muscle easily. I finally found my body's purpose: winter.

Now that we were married, I was starting to believe that Roy really liked me, ass and all, and perhaps with Allen and Bergmann to help boost my confidence, I could seduce my husband with newfound irresistible sexiness as someone perfectly equipped to survive *The Day After Tomorrow*.

---

6. A possible factor in Allen's Rule may be that cartilage growth partly depends on temperature; animals raised in cold climates tend to have lesser blood flow in their extremities, leading to less growth of bone and cartilage. We humans were equally susceptible to these effects for most of our existence, until we came up with coats and gloves and indoor heating.

I was maybe getting ahead of myself. After all, if Bergmann and Allen were still completely applicable today, Ukrainian supermodels wouldn't exist and neither would Pygmies, since they completely defy their environments. So do Dutch people.

When I studied in the Netherlands in college, I felt like a perpetual seven-year-old. Not only because I was always a little bit confused about what was going on around me, but because as an American of average height, I was minuscule compared to my Dutch counterparts. Most of my conversations took place looking squarely in my new compatriots' abdomens. Buying pants was also a problem. In fact, the Dutch are the tallest people in the world.

According to Bergmann and Allen, the Dutch should be short people, but they aren't. In 1860 the average height of a Dutch man was five foot five inches tall, three inches shorter than the average American man. But now the average Dutch male is well over six feet tall. Obviously the climate of the Netherlands hasn't changed drastically to mimic that of the Sahara—there had to be more at play to body size and shape than just climate.

Access to healthy food and quality medical care for all its citizens are two possible contributors to the countrywide growth spurt of the last 150 years, but a 2015 study published in *Proceedings B* found that it might actually be a product of natural selection. An analysis of 2,612 Dutch men and women over age forty-five, which focused on participants' height and number of offspring, found that taller men had more children on average than short and average-sized men. Not only that, women of average height had more children, but women who were taller had children at a faster rate, it is thought because they married later—possibly because of aesthetic preference.

Dr. Gert Stulp and his team of scientists who ran the study thought there might be a correlation between height and wealth, assuming those with more money had more resources for food and medical needs, but once the group was split into subgroups that controlled for income and education, the findings were the same: taller people have more children, at least in the Netherlands.

In America evolution seems to be taking us in a different direction. In a 2010 report published in *Proceedings of the National Academy of Sciences of the United States of America* (PNAS) titled "Natural Selection in a Contemporary Human Population," a sixty-year study that followed women involved in a 1948 study[7] and their descendants found that, as the gene pool progressed, women were likely to be shorter and stouter—American women, in Massachusetts at least, are shrinking.

---

7. The Framingham Heart Study.

I HAVE FAT

I've learned two important lessons in regard to world travel: a girl can absolutely live on brie alone, and English is the international language of travel. Wherever you are in the world, you'll usually find a sign in English to point you in the right direction or someone willing to take pity on you and speak to you in far better English than your broken their-language.

Russia hasn't received the memo. Other than the flight board, there wasn't a single sign in English or an English speaker anywhere in the Moscow airport, airline and airport staff included. We had eighteen hours to kill before our connecting flight to Tel Aviv, and it had taken us less than an hour to tour the duty-free shops for their sheer entertainment value. We learned that Vladimir Putin is a rock star to the airport-dwelling crowd: the clothing and souvenir shops, as well as all the vending machines littered throughout the airport, were filled with T-shirts of him—one of him horseback riding topless, one of him wrestling a bear, another one of him looking cool in a Hawaiian shirt and aviators, saying, "Welcome to Crimea" and other such gems. Putin's face adorned cigarette lighters, shot glasses, and souvenir bottles of vodka. So macabre entertainment we had aplenty, but what we had a hard time finding was something to eat.

We had learned through experience that ordering the vegetarian meal on discount Russian airlines meant getting chicken. Which didn't bother me, but Roy has slightly stricter standards on what counts as a vegetable. We figured we'd stay away from places that boasted meat in their title like Steak House, Burger King, and мясо, мясо, мясо! ("meat, meat, meat!"[1]).

We eventually found a kiosk that looked like the Russian equivalent of Subway and decided it was our safest bet. Through the combined alchemy of my phone, Google Translate, and a little game of charades, we eventually managed to order our food, with Roy getting a vegetable dish that consisted solely of potatoes and beets and me getting the Питания 1: from the photo it looked like a wrap filled with a hot dog and dill-mashed potatoes with mustard. By this point we were starving, and I felt confident that the hot-dog-potato-burrito would at least hold me over until we got to Israel.

I was feeling a little less than stellar by the time we landed. I didn't think much of it—I have a habit of feeling rotten after long flights and chalked it up to poor plane ventilation and a crappy immune system. On our first trip to Israel together I had contracted an eye infection on the flight and met his friends and family with one leaky eye swollen shut—I couldn't make a much worse impression this time.

It wasn't until an hour after we'd arrived at our rented apartment for the week that my body rebelled in a way typically seen in movies about demonic possession. At one point the sound of my violent heaving woke the baby upstairs. If I had any fluid left in my body, I would've cried too. And yet Roy, an army vet who usually wakes up at the drop of a pin, managed to sleep through it all. I alternated for a very long three hours between the bathroom and moaning curled up on the living room couch. But then I hit my crescendo and lost any humility left,

---

1.   I made that up.

along with any food I'd eaten in the past year or so. I woke Roy up. It looked like I was going to die, and I knew he'd want to say goodbye.

"Roy! You need to wake up!"

"Wha—" He looked up, slurring some syllables. Roy's never been much of a morning person. Especially at three a.m.

"I'm sick. I'm so sick," I managed to tell him, focusing on keeping all my orifices shut tight. "I need something. Do Israelis have Pepto?"

He didn't say anything, just staggered out of bed and got dressed (he remembers rushing, but I'm pretty sure it took him about six hours to tie his shoes), kissed my sweat-drenched forehead, and left. If he'd seen the bathroom, he wouldn't have come back.

Tel Aviv is a modern city, but it's not Manhattan with its twenty-four-hour Duane Reades on every corner. There was only one twenty-four-hour pharmacy around, and it wasn't walking distance. Roy took a cab, and since we hadn't exchanged enough money yet, he offered the driver American dollars and told him his wife was very sick. The driver wouldn't take his money and waited outside for Roy so he could take him back home.

Roy returned with the majority of a cracker aisle and a bunch of pills I couldn't read or pronounce with my crappy Hebrew. I continued to throw everything up, including the pills, and my *pill*, for the next three days, before I finally returned to normal. But there was an upside—I had lost five pounds.

We travel to Israel about once a year, usually in the scorching summer months, when Roy is off from his job as a college professor and most of his personal-training clients are out of town (ironically, it's his side job as a trainer that pays most of the bills, which says a lot about our culture: we pay people to build our bodies more than we pay people to expand our minds). Because of our wedding we were visiting in March, and while I was still reveling in the newfound knowledge that my body was a genetic winter warrior, Roy needed to get away from the thirty-degree New York spring.

As with every visit, the routine was the same: during the week we'd spend the day visiting his ninety-two-year-old grandmother, and in the evenings and weekends we'd hang out in Tel Aviv with his childhood friends. This often included eating out, but ironically no matter how much I eat in Israel, which is a lot, I always come home a few pounds thinner. It could be that there's just something about food that's not American that makes me thinner, but it could also be that the food in Israel is very produce heavy—almost every meal includes a fresh salad, and fruit smoothies are available on most city blocks. It's a fairly healthy culture, and up until recently, before American junk food became pervasive, their obesity levels reflected that.

Roy's grandma, Guta, had survived the Holocaust because she looked Aryan and spoke perfect German. Her family in Poland saw what was coming and sent her to school in Germany with fake documentation, where she spent the war hiding in plain sight. Aside from her youngest sister, who now lives in Brooklyn, she is the only survivor of her family. Her years there left their mark, one way being that she's obsessed with keeping up appearances. Still living in a fourth floor walk-up at ninety-two—which she says is how she got to be ninety-two—she spends an hour ironing her outfit, polishing her brooch, putting on makeup, and spraying her hair just to go to the grocery store on the corner to pick up milk and the newspaper, then return home, take it all off, and stay in.

Concerns over appearances rubbed off on Roy, whom she helped raise. Roy, like his grandma, dresses to send a message. It's because of this family concern with appearance that I wasn't all that surprised when Guta pointed out how much weight I'd gained almost as soon as I walked in the door. I'd been faithful to my nutritionist's reverse-dieting plan, but it had taken me a while to stop gaining, and Guta hadn't seen me since before most of my weight gain. Guta was someone who was always inclined to notice appearance and who called 'em like she saw 'em, but it's never easy hearing "You're fat." I seriously doubted that

Guta would understand if I told her that I'd done stupid things to my body over the years and that I'd gained weight as a result but I was trying to fix it by not dieting for a while and letting my body recover. So I just stood there and took it.

Of course, Guta didn't actually tell me directly. She told Roy to tell me.

"Guta says we're too fat; we need to lose weight," Roy said.

"Did she say 'we' or did she say 'I'?" I spoke enough Hebrew to know she hadn't referenced him at all in her comment.

He shrugged. "She said you, but she means both of us. I've gained weight too." It was a nice attempt to spare my feelings, but he knew I wasn't buying it.

"What is she saying now—verbatim, please."

He shook his head at me, as if to say, *It's your funeral.*

"You need to do more sport," she told me. "And you need to get pregnant."

"I can lose weight or I can get pregnant, Guta," I said, "but I can't do both." I knew her English wasn't good enough to catch most of that, and I knew Roy wouldn't translate it—so I felt okay being a bit saucy to my new grandmother-in-law.

So far I'd lost three days of my vacation to an impromptu colon cleanse, and now I was being told I was fat. The trip really couldn't have gotten much worse at that point, which was of course the perfect time to get my body fat measured at the Yair Lahav clinic, a training complex in Tel Aviv that caters to professional athletes and the super wealthy.

DEXA machines are mostly used by medical professionals. They look a lot like open MRIs and do a similar job—slowly scanning the makeup of your body. My mother gets one every year to measure her bone mass, thanks to early-onset osteoporosis. In the United States these tests would cost us a month's rent, but in Tel Aviv they're just a professional perk and the worst family tradition ever. The building has two stories, the first being a private gym where a handful of supertrainers work with clients, while the analytical staff on the second floor use state-of-the-art equipment to measure clients' body composition (fat, bone, and lean muscle mass) and metabolism.

I thought I was in really good shape the first time I came to Israel with Roy. When they handed me a body fat measurement of 32 percent, I started tearing up in the middle of the clinic, with Yair looking at me like I was crazy and Roy not sure whether to hug me or bury himself somewhere. I'd worked out constantly and ate so little, I deserved a lower number. I shouldn't have been made up of two-thirds person and one-third fat. Of course, then came the explanations that the ideal average for a thirty-year-old woman is between 25 and 30 percent and that I wasn't really that far off, and that I could just lose a few more pounds to get there.

In the two years since our first DEXA date, I'd gained forty pounds. I really didn't want to know what number would be waiting for me, but I was embracing the principle that knowledge is power. Awful, depressing power.

First, the bad news.

"It's too much fat," Eytan, the technician who did my DEXA analysis, said flatly. "You need to lose some fat."

Israelis are rather blunt by nature. They're just not an emotionally coddling sort of people. But they also don't take things personally. So, when an Israeli DEXA tech tells you that you need to lose fat, it's not a judgment—it's just a fact.

In English we say "I am fat" or "She is fat." The Hebrew equivalent means more "I have fat" or "She has fat." Weight is not a defining trait: it's not who you are; it's just something you have, which you can have less of or more of. I had more.

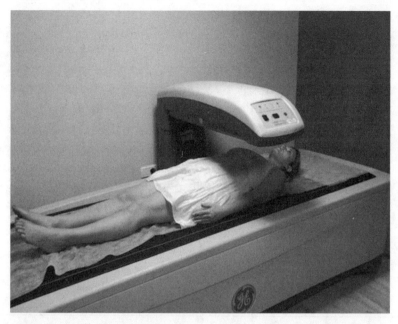

In the DEXA. I have enormous feet. I truly believe I was supposed to be much, much taller than I am.

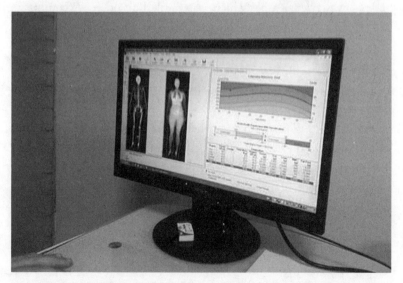

"It's too much fat," Eytan, the technician who did my DEXA analysis, said flatly. "You need to lose some fat."

"Yeah, I know," I said. "I'm trying."

I was 50.4 percent fat. A higher percentile of fat than I've ever had before. More fat than anything else in me. My only saving grace was that I also happened to have forty-two kilograms of lean muscle mass, which Eytan congratulated me on as being a lot for a woman my height, but to add insult to injury, my muscle mass had actually decreased since my last scan. I'd spent a not-so-small fortune on a CrossFit-loving personal trainer over the last year to get in wedding shape. I could deadlift my husband and kettlebell swing like a pro, and I'd come back home from the gym every other week proud of a new personal record, but I still lost muscle mass. Nothing in my world made sense. Roy was visibly concerned about my loss of muscle. It's the metabolic engine of the body—the more of it you have, the more calories you burn—so my metabolism had actually gone down. I had a feeling I wouldn't be renewing my personal-training package when we got back to the States.

According to my height-to-weight ratio my BMI—body mass index—was twenty-nine, which was borderline obese. According to the DEXA's much more specific measurements I was "only" overweight, with a true BMI of twenty-six, which I'd take, but still. I'd been working out intensely for the past year, I'd been disciplined about eating lean and healthy with very few exceptions, and yet I was made up of mostly fat. More of me was redundant in the world than not. I was a hypocrite, writing about health and fitness when I was probably fatter than most of my readers. And I was a failure, as a new wife who ballooned while Roy worked hard to maintain his superhero physique, and as a person, because I'd promised myself that I'd not be fat anymore, and I believed me. But mostly I was tired. Exhausted. I've been dieting since I was seven years old.

I still had one more test to undergo, but this one I was, though not quite looking forward to, curious to find out the results of. It was for my BMR (basal metabolic rate), which I'd tested before. It involves reclining for fifteen minutes and breathing into a mask that looks like something an apocalypse survivalist would have. Our bodies use oxygen as the main source of energy, and by measuring the difference between the amount of oxygen inhaled and the amount of oxygen and carbon dioxide exhaled (combined with other variables such as age, gender, weight, and body composition), the machine can accurately estimate how many calories one's body requires for its basic daily function—determining how many are needed to lose, maintain, or gain weight.

Eytan made me a latte and started going over my results. The last time I did the test was a year before, when my nutritionist sent me. At the time she had been concerned that I was burning around nine hundred calories a day—low for someone of my age and activity level. Alison had believed that years of deprivation had made my body adapt to surviving on very little food, which kept my metabolism very low. I'd spent the last year dedicated to her method of gradually eating more without gaining weight. It felt counterintuitive and uncomfortable, but I did it.

"Your BMR is 1,699. It's slightly higher than average for your age and size." Eytan looked as surprised as I was. "You probably could add a couple hundred to that for walking around during the day."

My BMR had nearly doubled in a year.

I had succeeded in fixing my metabolism, but I was still overweight. With my body finally functioning like a normal person's, I could finally lose the weight. I just had to figure out how. With a normal BMR I could restrict calories drastically and lose weight quickly, like back in my early dieting days. But that was what got me in trouble to begin with. I had to do this slowly, healthfully.

My weight was teetering on the BMI line between overweight and obese. I had a need-hate relationship with BMI: as the industry standard I had to use it daily at work, but I knew that it wasn't always accurate.

It was first developed in the mid-nineteenth century by a Belgian statistician named Adolphe Quetelet, but it was made famous by Ancel Keys—the same American scientist who ran the Minnesota Starvation Study—in the 1970s. BMI, calculated by dividing weight in kilograms by the square of height in meters, became the gold standard of weight classification for a long time. It's still commonly used by medical professionals, but many also dispute its validity because it doesn't take muscle or build into account. Two women who are each five foot six inches and weigh 160 pounds, for example, would both have a BMI of just over twenty-five, making them technically overweight, despite having different bone, muscle, and fat mass, with significantly different body-fat percentage. A very muscular man would be diagnosed as overweight or obese.

More recently a waist-to-height ratio has been lauded as a better measure of health, suggesting that one should aim to have a waist measurement that is half or lesser than their height in inches to prevent cardiovascular disease and metabolic syndrome. It's based on the idea that waist circumference is determined by the amount of fat tissue, and that stomach fat is more closely correlated with health issues than butt and hip fat. So those women who are five foot six inches and 160 pounds don't need to track down a BMI chart to find out if they're at risk for heart disease; they just need to measure their waist and see if it's 33 inches or less.

But biology hasn't anticipated modern culture. In a world that covets thigh gaps and bikini bridges, a thirty-three-inch waist might be perfectly healthy for someone with a broad build, but what's considered healthy isn't necessarily what's considered beautiful—which is why perfectly healthy people spend their lives feeling like crap.

It seems that when it comes to physical attraction, the hip-to-waist ratio is where it's at. In 2010, Johan Karremans, a psychologist at Radboud University in the Netherlands, published a paper in *Evolution and Human Behavior* titled "Blind Men Prefer a Low Waist-to-Hip

Ratio" (possibly the best scientific-study title ever). Karremans and his colleagues set out to find whether men's preference for certain female body types was something that was imprinted culturally or whether it was truly innate, as the consensus in the scientific community was— that men who are attracted to women, regardless of their country, culture, or race, prefer women with a low waist-to-hip ratio, meaning with a waist significantly narrower than the hips.

In the age of globalization, culture is increasingly homogenized, and especially in the west, the media promotes a fairly standardized model of the female form. It could be that the preference for an hourglass figure is really a byproduct of that: men and women are bombarded with the same images, telling women what they should look like and men what they should look for.

Karremans and his crew set up a series of mannequins with varying waist-to-hip ratios, ranging from very low (notable difference between the waist and hips) to very high (fuller waist with slight increase to hips), all within normal range for women. They then asked men who'd been blind since birth to pick which body shape was most attractive based on touch. Virtually all chose the mannequin with the lowest ratio. Men are hardwired to prefer women with small waists.

The evolutionary theory is that this "ideal" ratio was indicative of health and fertility, therefore appealing to a man's primal instinct to propagate.[2] The theory is backed by various studies, like the 2007 report

---

2. Men haven't been wholly ignored as objects of desire by the scientific community, although they certainly haven't received the same amount of attention as women. A man's shoulder-to-waist ratio has been found to convey similar information about their reproductive/genetic quality. You guessed it. Broad shoulders, tiny waists tested better when it came to attractiveness.

in *Evolution and Human Behavior,*[3] which found that lower body fat has positive effects on brain development, and that women with lower ratios, as well as their children, have significantly higher cognitive test scores. As crazy as it sounds, the conclusion is that men lust after 36-24-36 women because they're likelier to provide them with smart children.

---

3. Former assistant surgeon general William D. Lassek, MD, and Steven J. C. Gaulin, PhD, the men behind these particular findings, also coauthored a book called *Why Women Need Fat.* I haven't read it, but it sounds delightful.

FOUR

FEED A COLD, STARVE A FETUS

"In six months."

People started asking us when we were going to have a baby around the same time we cut our wedding cake. We'd always tell them we'd start trying in six months. Whenever it was they asked, we'd tell them, "In six months."

Roy and I had actually started talking about having kids not long after he gave me a toothbrush and asked me to be his girlfriend. It was something we were going to do in the future, like owning a summer home (or an actual home) or going to Italy or having a dishwasher. But my bout of food poisoning when we were in Israel screwed with my birth control, and we needed to decide what to do, what kind of contraception we'd use until I could get back on track—if we even wanted to get back on track. I was thirty-two. My mother started trying to get pregnant at my age, and it took her two years, which didn't leave me much time for a worry-free second pregnancy if I wanted one. Was my biblical plague–level food poisoning actually divine intervention? Maybe it was time. Getting pregnant isn't complicated in theory, but

I'd spent all of my sexually active life trying not to get pregnant. It was uncharted territory.

I didn't tell Roy right away that I was thinking that maybe our six months were up. There were moments when I looked at him and he was so sweet and goofy and beautiful that I was scared of how much I loved him, how much it would hurt me if I lost him. In these random moments in time I forgot that he wasn't just some guy I had a crush on but my husband. What if I brought up this big, serious life change, and instead of wrapping his arms around me, he threw them up in the air with an exasperated sigh and disappointed glare? "You've been great, but . . ."

I have a bad habit of bringing up important topics like prenups, mortgages, and gene sharing in public places, casually. It's a defense mechanism, wholly inappropriate, like taking a date to a restaurant to break up with them so they won't make a scene. But it's a method that's never failed me: I say something at the worst possible time, and Roy just pretends that it's completely normal. For the baby-making discussion, I chose Petco. I didn't really choose; it just felt so wrong that it was right.

Roy's wedding gift to me was an IOU for a puppy. He didn't actually want a dog, but I'd grown up with dogs and missed having a belly to scratch and someone to lick away tears. As soon as our flight back from our honeymoon landed, we went to a shelter to window-shop our options. Right as we walked in, one of the volunteers thrust a corgi/beagle mix into my arms, and I knew that we needed to keep her. One simply does not browse for puppies. As the volunteers checked our references and ran Roy's credit card, we decided we would name her Inez. Inez the Bitch—after the terrible girlfriend in *Midnight in Paris*—and it just seemed so perfect at the time.

We jokingly referred to her as our practice baby: we'd only been practicing for a few months, but so far she'd destroyed everything nice we owned and made it reasonably clear that she wasn't particularly fond of us, so it seemed like we were ready for the real thing.

"Do you think we should get Inez a harness for running? I don't want to pull on her neck," I asked. The weather was warming up, and we were planning on taking our morning cardio dates outside.

"Sure."

"Do you want to use condoms?" I slipped in.

"On Inez?"

"No, I mean, I'm not on the pill anymore, so how do you want to go about preventing a tiny human from happening?"

"Condoms are fine," he said.

"What about not using condoms? We could use the rhythm method, or not?"

"Kim, do you want to get pregnant?" He catches on quick.

"I don't not want to get pregnant," I answered. That was true. I wasn't quite ready to start charting my temperatures and ordering him to bed around ovulation. But I was also willing to let nature take its course and see what happened.

"If you want to get pregnant, we can get pregnant." He looked at me reassuringly. He'd already told me that it was my call, at my comfort. I just looked through the cans of dog food. I had a whole line of points to make, and he was being far too agreeable.

"My doctor said it should take around three months for the pill to cycle out once I'm off, so maybe we just use these three months to enjoy hormone-free sex and then let nature take its course."

"When's the best time of year to have a baby?" he asked, practical as ever. "Maybe we should time it? I'm assuming it's ideal to have one when the weather's nice outside."

"Well, the doctor said it could take up to a year for a healthy couple to get pregnant, so I don't know that we can really time it." My ob-gyn had been reminding me every Pap exam since I turned thirty that I was getting old and needed to have a baby immediately. I maybe needed to find a new doctor. "Plus, I hear it sucks having a newborn no matter what time of year it is." My father always said that having a baby doesn't really have an upside until they're about six months old and can interact with you. My mom declared that I was her best friend from the moment she knew she was pregnant. I believed my dad.

"Okay, so let's get pregnant."

"Okay," I said. "We should also pick up some wet food."

After we got home and lavished Inez with all sorts of unreciprocated attention—because she hates us—I downloaded *What to Expect Before You're Expecting* on my Kindle and read it in a couple of hours.

It was a big decision, the biggest decision, and I wasn't 100 percent sure that I was as ready for it as I'd thought. The book stressed the importance of being at a healthy weight while trying to conceive. I was maintaining steadily at my wedding weight—unsure what the right way to go was now that I had "fixed" my broken metabolism—but I was still carrying most of the weight I'd gained. The book made it pretty clear that if I was selfish enough to conceive while overweight, I would be putting myself and my baby at risk. I'd be at higher risk for preeclampsia, gestational diabetes, a C-section, and a bunch of other scary things. I've never had any health problems; even at my heaviest my blood tests and physicals were nearly textbook perfect, so I decided that I would just eat clean and healthy and in moderately smaller portions until I knew I was pregnant. That way I'd be losing until I was supposed to be gaining. A compromise between my body and me.

When I woke up the next morning Roy was already up, sitting on the couch doing research for a book he'd been working on. After "Good morning," he said out of the blue, "I've been thinking about our conversation yesterday . . . What about your weight?"

"What about my weight?" I replied, defensively.

"You want to lose weight; that's going to be harder after you have a baby. What happens if you get pregnant now and you find yourself stuck at a weight you're unhappy with?"

I can't remember a time I was actually happy about my weight, I thought, but I didn't want him to realize that being happy wasn't an actual option for me. It wasn't about being able to diet after having a baby that I was worried about; it was that my research into baby making really drove home the fact that I needed to lose weight to have a healthy pregnancy. I had been selfish by letting my weight get so out of hand. It was unfair to my future family. I wasn't even pregnant and I was already a terrible mother. I started crying, so I did the dishes to cover up the sniffles.

When Roy realized what was happening, he apologized.

"I'm sorry. I don't know what I said, but I'm sorry."

"You just said I was too fat to get pregnant!"

I was not rational about my weight. I could be rational about everything else in my life, but no matter how much research I've done, no matter how many articles I've written, I could never be rational about my body.

"I didn't say that. I didn't mean to say that. I just want you to be happy, I don't want you to spend your life frustrated about your weight. We can get pregnant today if you want."

"No, we can't; I'm not ovulating."

"Okay," he said. "When you are." He was being so sweet, but I was still too fat to have his baby.

My mother has always said that pregnancy was the best time of her life. All six months of it—I was born three months early. Other than her advanced age (back in the early eighties, thirty-four was considered geriatric in the obstetrics ward), there were no signs that she would have an at-risk pregnancy. The fact that she didn't gain a single pound didn't set off any alarm bells.

"I hope you have a baby just like you. You were always the best baby," she gloated when I called to tell her about our decision. "You never cried in the middle of the night, and I lost twelve pounds right after you were born."

The truth is that I did wake up in the middle of the night, as my dad would remind me, as he was the one who would pick me up and feed me. My mom was apparently a very sound sleeper. I'd been hearing the story of my mom's miraculous pregnancy weight loss my entire life, and just figured she was a biological anomaly. I'd always hoped I'd inherit her magical metabolism and also leave the hospital a dress size smaller.

Optimal baby-making conditions seemed to be an ongoing theme in my life. At work we were gearing up to publish a book about epigenetics, the premise being that one can shut off their fat genes. I was uncomfortable with the idea that we were painting a picture of evil genes lurking inside our bodies, but it was my job, and I did the research I was asked to, which is when I came across a study of the infamous 1944 Dutch famine, also known as the Dutch Hunger Winter.

At the end of World War II, the Netherlands was cut off from outside trade of food and fuel by the Germans, and since it was winter and there were no crops, food quickly became scarce. Between November 1944 and late spring of 1945, 4.5 million people endured extreme malnutrition in what came to be known as the Dutch Hunger Winter. One of the starving was fifteen-year-old Audrey Hepburn, who was Belgian but living in the Netherlands at the time. Her body never recovered from the effects of the famine, leaving her with a small, frail build—a look that ironically made her a beauty icon in her adult life. Hepburn can be considered lucky; it's estimated that twenty-two thousand people starved to death in that bleak period of Dutch history, as government rations for adults were reduced from one thousand calories a day to under six hundred. People resorted to eating tulip bulbs, family pets, and even furniture to stay alive.

While all this was happening, researchers at the Academic Medical Center in Amsterdam took the opportunity to learn more about the effects of famine on pregnant women. Because they were pregnant, they were allotted nine hundred calories a day—roughly half of the recommended intake for pregnant women, but significantly more than the rest of the adult population; 923 of the 1,116 women recruited carried full term, and they and their children were studied over the next forty years. It was one of the very first studies in epigenetics—the study of gene expression[1]—and one of the first studies that illustrated a link between external influences and metabolic gene expression.

The researchers found that women who had a normal diet for the majority of their pregnancy before the famine started and were exposed to a period of malnutrition only in the last trimester were likely to have underweight babies, and those babies grew up to be small adults, with significantly lower overweight and obesity rates than the general population.

On the other hand, women who experienced famine in the beginning of their pregnancy but returned to proper nourishment at the end gave birth to babies of a normal weight. Interestingly, those babies went on to have a much higher than average rate of obesity later in life. The results of the study tell us that, depending on the stage of pregnancy, in-utero nutrition can affect the child's lifelong metabolism, making them more or less likely to be overweight in adulthood.[2]

I started asking my mom about her diet during her pregnancy. My parents had tried so long to conceive that once she was pregnant, she was paranoid that she'd do something wrong; she cut everything unnatural and processed out of her diet. My mom started eating organic before organic was a thing.

---

1.   Epigenetics is the study of how outside influences can affect our genes. Certain genes can be activated, left dormant, or suppressed—effectively switched on or off—affecting things like disease, height, metabolism, etc. The field of epigenetics is still in its infancy but will likely enable us in the not-too-far future to control various genetic attributes, like babies' eye color or skin shade, putting it at the forefront of not just science but moral philosophy.
2.   That doesn't mean that the first group's results were "good." Please don't starve your fetus. Better yet, consult a nutritionist.

"You know, I cut so much out of my diet that I wasn't eating much at all. Maybe your weight issues are my fault." My mother is always eager to take responsibility for anything that is wrong with me. But she wasn't starving during her pregnancy like one of the Dutch women. She didn't eat enough to gain weight, but I was born exactly the right weight for a thirty-week preemie: three pounds. It's likely that I was getting my share of calories from her fat stores, which is why she lost twelve pounds right after I was born. I'm always on the hunt for excuses to pin my weight issues on, but I wasn't going to blame my mother for this one.

WHOSE LINE IS IT ANYWAY?

Food. Sex. And. According to my wise best friend, Anna, all men are made up of a simple trifecta of priorities. The "and" is what changes from man to man. For her boyfriend it's cars. For my husband it's superheroes—mostly in the form of comics, but superhero movies are still a matter of utmost importance in our home. When the most recent installment of the Marvel Cinematic Universe is announced, we buy tickets as far in advance as possible so that we can reserve seats on opening night in the exact middle of the theater. Once tickets are purchased, Roy starts making a list of the candy he will indulge in during the film. For a man who sports a permanent six-pack, my husband can put away an astonishing amount of corn syrup in one sitting. For the second *Avengers* movie our (his) menu would include: Sour Patch Kids, Riesen chocolates, Skittles, Starburst minis (because the full-size candies have gelatin and he's a vegetarian), and M&Ms. I'm not really a sweets person, but I'll usually pick on a couple of pieces, which I did when we went to see the movie. But it all tasted weird. Too sweet. Kind of metallic.

I whispered to Roy during a Scarlet Witch scene that something was wrong with the candy, but he quickly shushed me.

The next morning I drank a glass of juice with breakfast, which tasted weird too. Something was wrong with my mouth. My period was still a few days off, but I had stocked up on cheap pregnancy tests from China. I couldn't imagine ever needing fifty pregnancy tests, but for $11, I figured it couldn't hurt to have them around.

Negative.

My doctor had told me that it would take a few months for my body to regulate after going off of the pill, so I wasn't surprised. I'd been pill-free for less than a month.

The next morning, same thing. My juice was off. As was the salad I ate for lunch; it tasted like they'd poured sugar on the cucumbers. I took a nap midday and chalked up my exhaustion to unconscious procrastination.

The day my period was due I figured I'd start the morning with another pregnancy test. I'd still have forty-eight at my disposal. I dunked the tiny stick in a plastic cup of urine and set it aside while I went about my normal morning routine. I took a shower, brushed my teeth, and took a quick glance at the stick on the way out of the room.

"Is this a line?" I said, tumbling out of the bathroom, disheveled and shell-shocked, shoving my urine-soaked stick in Roy's face just as he walked in the door from walking Inez.

From the moment we decided that we'd forgo birth control and let nature take its course, I had a plan of how I'd tell Roy the news. I would wait to tell him, not too long, maybe a few days, while I gathered up onesies and other baby paraphernalia that represented our life together: a onesie from NYU, where he was getting his master's degree when we met; a bib in Hebrew, Roy's native language (I had started taking lessons when we got engaged so we could raise our children in a bilingual home, a goal I was perpetually failing at accomplishing); an *I ♥ New York* toddler-sized T-shirt, and something with our dog's face on it, because, after all, Inez is our first baby together, even if she hates us. Then I would bundle it all together with a pregnancy test and voilà: the gift of fatherhood. I was secretly hoping it would all go down in June so I could give it to him as a Father's Day gift.

Instead, I announced my pregnancy in the least romantic way I could have. Barefoot, towel turban flopping to one side, and a trail of footprint-shaped puddles behind me.

He held the pregnancy test, inspecting it with care, while using his other hand to unleash Inez.

"Yes, but let's not get ahead of ourselves. It's very light. It could be a false positive," he responded. Pragmatic. Not the reaction I'd fantasized about.

Based on the nine thousand or so YouTube videos of candid pregnancy reveals I'd watched in preparation, I was hoping he'd sweep me up in an embrace with tears in his eyes. Roy was the romantic one; it was his job to get choked up and tell me how happy he was. Maybe he wasn't happy.

I proceeded to dunk several more tests in my fresh cup of morning pee. All with the same result, a faint pink line.

"Yeah, it's probably nothing," I said, pouring my almond-milk latte down the drain.

The pink line got darker over the next few days, and as it did our priorities changed. But first, I wanted to tell my parents.

Father's Day was out, but Mother's Day was just around the corner. We were planning on heading out to Long Island to take my mom out for a Mother's Day lunch. Roy thought we should wait until we were further along, but I assured him that was just for friends. Parents should be told right away. "Plus," I said, "if something goes wrong, I'm going to need my mom."

It took all my willpower not to tell her on the phone.

"Hi, honey, when are you coming out on Sunday?" she asked.

"I made reservations for two o'clock," I told her, "but I figured Roy and I would come out earlier, and we could spend some time at home before we go out." I didn't want to tell her she was going to be a grandmother in a restaurant.

"Sure," she said. "When are you due?"

"What?" *January 14. How did she know?*

"For your period. When are you due?" My family isn't really big on boundaries. My cycle and sex life are discussed as nonchalantly as the weather or the most recent episode of *Criminal Minds*. It was a running joke that it doesn't matter what time of month it is, every time I set foot on Long Island I get my period. My dad simply picks me up at the train station and drives directly to the drugstore without any need for discussion.

"Oh, sorry, I was distracted by Inez . . . Thursday."

"Well, I hope you don't get it." I'd like to say that this kind of comment was unique, but it wasn't. When Roy and I moved in together, my father bought us a windowsill herb garden as a housewarming gift. My mother crocheted us a gender-neutral green baby blanket (when I unwrapped it, Roy stared at it for a moment, then said, "I can't put my finger on it, but I get the sense your mom is trying to tell us something"). Then for our first holidays in our new home, she got us a gift subscription to *Parents* magazine, so we could "study." Now that we had a few months of marriage under our belt, she couldn't understand why we didn't already have three kids.

After I hung up with my mom I walked Inez over to a card store, where she promptly eviscerated a little stuffed animal and I had to buy it along with my card. I didn't get a Mother's Day card, just a plain blank one with a cover that said "You're the Best."

When we got back to the apartment I added "Mom" to the front of the card with a thick Sharpie that matched the ink and wrote inside:

Which is why you're being promoted to grandmother.
Please report for your new position in January of 2016.
With love,
Kim, Roy, and the bundle of baby cells in my uterus

Roy and I held hands the whole two-hour train ride to my parents' house, enjoying our secret while it lasted. I thought my mom would know as soon as I stepped off the train. I was five minutes pregnant, but I felt like it was written all over my face. She didn't.

My parents being my parents, we had to stop at two different places to pick up some things they needed, and it took us an extra hour and change to get home. By the time we got to their house, I couldn't wait anymore.

"Mom, do you want your cards?"

"I would love them."

I looked at my dad, indicating he should hand over his card first, but he didn't get the hint, so Roy handed her ours.

She read it and then looked up at me.

"Really?" she whispered.

"Really." I shook my head and started crying.

"This is the best gift . . ."

"We decided to go with something homemade this year," I said, my mom's arms already around me.

"Brian, did you read the card?" Roy asked, and handed it to my father.

He read it, then reread it. Nothing. For about five minutes, while my mom was talking up a storm, he just looked at the card, then at us, then at the card again. I wasn't sure if he was happy, if he was upset, if he was in shock. I didn't get any response from him, which made me sad. How could you not be overjoyed about being a grandfather?

Then he said, with an expression that started as deadpan but ended up as a big happy smile across his face, "I thought you were going to wait to have sex."

My mom had described to me, in detail, repeatedly, all the foods I could and could not have now that I was pregnant. I had changed my diet completely, happily, as soon as that line turned pink. I had no problem nixing anything with artificial colors or sweeteners, which we didn't eat much of anyway. I added four hundred calories to my daily allowance, not because there's a need for an increase in calories during the first trimester but because I was afraid my regular, diet-conscious eating habits were too minimal to make a new human. I'd deal with being fat later; the next nine months were about the baby, and I loved it.

For the first time in years, maybe my whole life, I wasn't self-conscious about my body. Nothing had changed; I just didn't think about whether I looked thin enough. I was pregnant; if anyone scoffed at my size (which no one ever had, at least not to my face, but I was always acutely afraid someone would), I could proudly announce that I wasn't fat, I was with child. Postmeal bloat would no longer be referred to as my food baby—it was my real baby.

My friends had all given their embryos cute little names like Chili, or Kiwi, or Bean. Roy and I decided on *Soomsoom*, Hebrew for sesame seed (on account of it being that size at the time). We also decided that for the time being, Soomsoom would be a boy. My family had a striking lack of males; statistically we were due for a boy in the gene pool. And I didn't have much in regard to pregnancy symptoms; I'd heard that girls were a little harder on the system than boys. We still had weeks and weeks till we could find out if we were right about Soomsoom's sex, but in the meantime we referred to Soomsoom as a he because having a pronoun made him feel more real. A son. We were going to have a son, who might also be a daughter. We really didn't care. Well, Roy cared a little; he thought a boy first and then a girl, so she could have an older brother to look after her. That, and he already decided on Soomsoom's first Halloween costume, which he called dibs on: baby Kal-El in a stroller decked out like his rocket ship, and Roy as daddy Jor-El. Superman was Roy's first-ever Halloween costume when he came to the United States, and he thought it'd make for a nice symmetry. He was going to make a great dad.

For Soomsoom we were ready to do all sorts of things that we swore we never would, like leave New York City. I grew up in the suburbs and couldn't wait to leave. I swore I would never live in the land of big-box stores again. I prided myself on not having owned a car since I was a teenager, that I used my legs as my main form of transportation. That I lived my life in the most exciting, bustling metropolis in the world. But for Soomsoom I wanted the world of my childhood. Long Island was made for kids. Good schools, parks, sports, museums, beaches—I wanted him to live where childhood was taken seriously, where it was safe to ride his bike down the street and he could run from one backyard sprinkler to the next and come home when the street lights went on. Those were things I didn't realize I loved about my childhood until I was a grown-up.

Roy grew up in Tel Aviv, which basically looks like Queens with a Santa Monica–esque beach. He'd never lived in a house, he didn't drive a car, weekends with my parents surrounded by trees and stillness drove him crazy—but he too wanted the idyllic life Long Island offered for our baby. We spent our nights looking at houses and researching school districts and our weekends with a Realtor, looking at different neighborhoods. We found a perfect little starter home in a sweet, quaint town just forty minutes from the city by train, and got approved for a mortgage. The commute wouldn't be too hard, and there were sidewalks for Soomsoom to play on and a small walkable village nearby for our sanity. For Soomsoom we would give up the city life we loved, happily. Roy started looking for better-paying jobs. I took on more freelance work. We would have less time to enjoy our lives, to enjoy each other, but our son would have everything we could give him, or her.

My mother always said that she'd never felt better than when she was pregnant—not only did she miraculously lose weight, but the life-long pain she'd had from her acute scoliosis cleared up, and she *finally* had boobs.

I've always thought my mother was beautiful. She was small, with lean arms and legs and beautiful red hair and dark brown eyes. As she's aged her auburn hair has turned to a strawberry blonde, with sections of white-blonde highlights. But my mother has always hated the way she looks. Since my earliest days she has waved off compliments. "I look like a monster," she says, always. The severe scoliosis she's suffered from since childhood has gotten worse over time. Her spine has such an acute curve that some of her vertebrae have fused together. It's pushed her internal organs forward, making her stomach pronounced. She always wears a pained expression, even when she smiles. She tells me I don't see her how she really looks, because I love her too much. But that's not true. She doesn't love herself enough.

I didn't want history to repeat itself. I was pregnant now, and that made me feel like the clock was ticking; I needed to find peace with my body. It was going to change, it was going to get fatter, and the amount of fat I have could not be my priority any longer. I was making a person. A person who was going to look to me and want to know how they should feel about themselves. I didn't want to screw that up.

There was a part of me that secretly wished that my baby was not a she, because the world is so much harder on girls. The pressure to be everything, to be smart but also to be beautiful, ambitious but also sup-portive of everyone else, carefree but thoughtful, full of personality and gravitas but also in great shape—it's a tightrope that I've fallen from on many occasions. The feminist in me wants to say, "Fuck the tightrope," but the truth is I don't know who I would be without it; my whole life has been centered around my performance. I suppose there are different battles men fight, but I honestly don't think they're as hard to balance.

If Soomsoom did turn out to be a boy, how could I teach him to respect women's bodies when I didn't respect mine? How could I not bequeath him, or her, the burden of self-disappointment and self-loathing? How could I make sure it ended with me?

In the first two weeks of my known pregnancy, I'd lost three pounds despite my calorie increase. I assumed it was because I'd cut wine and lattes out of my diet. I also had zero symptoms: while other new pregnant women on the Internet were bemoaning their morning sickness and extreme exhaustion I felt exactly the way I always did. It became nerve-racking once I'd started to bleed.

I didn't have an appointment until our eighth week, but I was convinced something was wrong. I asked if the doctor would see me and take a blood test to make sure everything was okay.

I had decided to switch doctors and go with a friend's ob-gyn ever since mine became baby crazed and started harassing me about getting knocked up every time I saw her. My new doctor, Dr. Shim, ushered us into his office and was very welcoming, though he mostly seemed like he'd seen far too many hysterical pregnant women to take me seriously.

"Honestly, if you're going to miscarry, you're going to miscarry. There's nothing we can do about it at this stage. It just means that there was something wrong with the baby. But I don't see any reason why you would. You're healthy. Lots of women spot."

"Should I be adjusting my exercise routine?" I'd been nervous about keeping up with my normal routine, which consisted of three days of strength training and three to four spin classes a week. Roy said it was fine, but I needed a doctor to tell me. I'd been avoiding working out since I found out I was pregnant.

"No, you can keep doing what you're doing."

"I lift heavy," I told him.

"As long as you're used to your workouts, there's no reason you shouldn't continue through your first trimester. In a few months, as your balance changes, you'll have to make some adjustments."

"It gets really hot in the spin room," I said.

"It's fine, really."

He ushered me over to a nurse who took my blood and gave me a "So, you're going to have a baby" care package full of prenatal vitamin samples and a list of things I should and shouldn't do while pregnant.

The results took forever. After five days the nurse finally called. "You have a hypoactive thyroid; you need to see an endocrinologist right away," she said in the same tone of voice as she might have said "Your shoe's untied" or "You've got some schmutz on your face."

"I know," I said. "My doctor said it wasn't an issue."

"Thyroid issues that aren't an issue in normal life are an issue when you're pregnant," she told me. "Ideally, you'd be medicated before you try to conceive."

My old doctor had never mentioned anything about my thyroid and pregnancy.

Now that my new one had raised a red flag, I couldn't stop seeing information about hypothyroidism in pregnancy everywhere I looked, probably because I spent all day looking it up on Google. There were articles and case studies and message boards all focused around women who had an untreated subclinical hypothyroid, and how they not only had a harder time conceiving but many went on to miscarry. And for those who didn't there was an increased risk of neurological development disorders.

I called more than a dozen endocrinologists; all told me that their wait time for an appointment was over a month away. The one Dr. Shim had referred me to told me in May that they wouldn't be able to see me until October.

"I'll be six months pregnant by then!"

"There are a lot of pregnant women in New York," the receptionist informed me.

Finally I gave up and called Dr. Shim's office and told them I couldn't get an appointment. He made a few calls and found a doctor who'd fit me in as a favor the following week.

The only people I could admit I was pregnant to were doctors and strangers I'd never see again. I found myself working the words "I'm" and "pregnant" into conversations with random customer service reps and cashiers because it was so unreal. I relished filling out my new endocrinologist's information sheet. Preexisting conditions: pregnant. Medications: prenatal vitamin. Reason for visit: I'm pregnant! / my TSH levels are high.

Dr. Birnbaum was a soft-spoken, thorough older gentleman. I expected him to take a look at my lab work, acknowledge the fact that I needed medicine, and write something up. But he wanted to weigh me and measure me (which is how I learned that I'd been living a lie and was actually an inch taller than I always thought I was, which lowered my BMI by a whole point, so there's that). He gave me a full physical, gently prodding at my glands. He seemed embarrassed to have to give me a naked physical, and I was embarrassed because he was embarrassed.

"You're overweight," he said.

"I know," I replied.

"You should have been medicated years ago for your thyroid."

Dr. Birnbaum showed me pictures of what a normal thyroid looked like, like a butterfly, kind of. And then he showed me sonogram pictures of my own, a pockmarked rock. My thyroid was covered in scar tissue, misshapen from years of inflammation caused by an untreated autoimmune disease doctors had been telling me since high school was no big deal.

My doctor had given me the lowest dose possible of synthetic thyroid hormones to hold me over, but my new endocrinologist told me that I needed much, much more than that to hopefully bring my TSH levels down to an appropriate level. Hopefully we caught it early enough and Soomsoom was going to be okay.

I started bleeding three days later.

WHAT TO EXPECT WHEN YOU'RE LOSING YOUR BABY

In movies, miscarriages play out like this: our protagonist awakens from a peaceful sleep to find that her nightgown—always a nightgown—is soaked through with blood. She wails and clutches her blood-soaked nightgown. She's sad the next morning. Sometimes she's in the hospital. But things get better immediately after. She gets over it and is back to being her smiling self. She goes shopping with friends for new nightgowns.

That's not how it happened with Soomsoom. I was sitting in a café, finishing up my writing for the afternoon, the same café in which Roy had asked me to be his girlfriend almost four years earlier. I stepped in the bathroom before packing up. Since day one of my pregnancy I made a point of using whatever bathroom was near me before embarking on the bathroomless great outdoors. There was blood. A lot of blood. I knew.

I washed up and texted Roy: I'm miscarrying. Getting on the subway. Please call dr.

A calm, stoic automaton, I got on the subway, walked home, went up the stairs, and went to the bathroom to check if I was still bleeding. It seemed to have stopped. I rubbed Inez's belly for a few minutes, who seemed genuinely happy to see me for possibly the first time.

"The doctor told us to come in right away," Roy relayed. "The nurse didn't seem concerned; it's probably fine."

"It's not," I said. "Let's go."

I didn't really like Dr. Shim; he didn't at all seem concerned when I told him that my pregnancy symptoms had faded to almost nothing and when I told him that the baby was measuring behind at our week-eight ultrasound. So I was relieved that there was another doctor on duty. A woman I'd never met.

"I'm sorry. I didn't shave my legs," I said. "I didn't think I'd be here today."

"Don't worry; I didn't shave mine either." She smiled.

"Me either," Roy chimed in.

"So we're all hairy," the doctor said while prepping the ultrasound machine. I wish I'd seen her from the beginning; maybe she would have taken me seriously when I said I thought there was something wrong with Soomsoom.

"I started bleeding. I'm just scared something is wrong," I said almost apologetically.

"I know. Let's see what's going on. You're going to feel a little pressure."

The ultrasound wand entered my body and Soomsoom appeared. He was bigger than the last time, but the flicker of his heart was gone. The doctor moved the wand around looking, but I knew she wouldn't find it. He was only measuring six weeks and two days. His heart had stopped before I had even seen the endocrinologist.

"I'm so sorry," she said. The nurse started rubbing my stubbly calf, trying to comfort me. Roy squeezed my shoulder. There were so many people touching me in a very small room.

"Okay," I said. "What do I do now?"

"Well, you could wait to miscarry naturally. Since you're bleeding already there's a good chance your cervix is already preparing for that, but it can take a few weeks to complete. I can give you a prescription that will bring on a natural miscarriage faster, or you could have a surgery."

"A D&C?" A good friend of mine had one. I remembered her telling me how she'd gone to the doctor for a regular appointment, found out that her baby had stopped growing, and was rushed in for a D&C without time to process what had happened. I didn't want to wake up and not be pregnant; I didn't want surgery. I wanted to still be pregnant with Soomsoom.

"Yes, a D&C. We would arrange for you to go into the hospital, and in most cases you're released directly afterward," the doctor said.

"No surgery. Can you give me the prescription and I'll wait to see if I need to fill it?" I wanted to do it as naturally as possible.

"Yes. I'm so sorry," she said, again. "I know this baby was wanted."

This baby was wanted. No one had acknowledged that yet, not me, not Roy. We had gotten pregnant easily, surprisingly easily, and it was sort of a high-five moment. We were planning to uproot our entire lives, but neither of us had actually said, "I want this baby" or "I'm so happy we're having this baby." And those were the words that shook me from my apathy. Roy and I had been so careful to keep each other in check, always phrasing Soomsoom's future in question form. We promised we'd allow ourselves to get excited once we hit the second trimester, like we were supposed to, but the truth was that we were already excited. Our baby was wanted.

I started sobbing, and apologizing for sobbing, and as I did everyone else in the tiny exam room seemed to want to touch me, to soothe me—I was the star of the miscarriage show.

"When will we be able to try again?" Roy asked. Army man, problem solver: take action, mourn later. It's how he deals with things. I didn't want to be pregnant with a new baby—I wanted to still be pregnant with my baby.

"You'll need to wait for your cycle to come back, and then I'd like for you to let two menses pass. After the miscarriage is complete, I will monitor your hormone levels and wait for your HCG to go back to zero, and then you can start again."

I nodded.

"I'm sorry," she said again. "We need your thyroid to be well under control before you get pregnant again."

I nodded.

The nurse, still rubbing my calves, looked like she was going to cry. She'd told me before that she'd been doing this for forty years, and I wondered if this part ever got easier. "If you need to talk to someone, you can call me here," she said.

I couldn't imagine calling the doctor's office to cry with the nurse, but I appreciated her warmth.

They left quietly, and I stood up and looked at Roy.

"I'm sorry," he said, over and over again, and he held me. I didn't know what to say back. It wasn't his fault. It was mine. My body wasn't good enough. My metabolism killed our baby.

"Are you okay?" I finally said.

"No, not really."

"Yeah."

"We'll wait the two months, and then we'll try again. We'll have another Soomsoom," Roy said.

"It won't be Soomsoom; it will be someone else," I said. I wondered what it would be like to have sex with the sole purpose of making a baby. I didn't want that, but I could see myself becoming obsessed with tracking ovulation dates and cervical mucus. It seemed like a crappy way to make a baby. Not out of love but out of a sense of failure.

We had tickets that night to see *Jersey Boys* on Broadway with my parents. It was their anniversary gift, and they'd been looking forward to it for months. I didn't want to ruin everyone's night, so I rallied. We took them out to a famous Italian restaurant off Times Square before the show and tried to pretend everything was fine. They saw right through us, more so me, and we ended up telling them as soon as we sat down.

My mother ordered me a martini. "Drink this," she said. She told me that she'd had a miscarriage once, which I never knew, when she was nineteen, while she was married to her first husband. It was early, earlier than mine. She wasn't upset about it, and one day I wouldn't be either.

My father didn't say much. He doesn't do well with the hard emotional stuff, but he put his arm around me as we walked to the theater. When Frankie Valli's daughter died in the show, I looked over and he was tearing up. I'd only seen him cry twice before: when my mom was in the hospital and when his sister died.

I woke up every morning and cried. Roy sat next to me and held me until I was ready to face the day. The miscarriage didn't happen naturally like I hoped it would. I waited for the bleeding to get heavy so I could say goodbye and let it be over. It didn't.

I had nightmares. One night I dreamt that I had forgotten to tell people I had miscarried, and my mother was throwing me a baby shower. I rushed to tell them that I wasn't pregnant anymore, but no one would believe me. I woke up confused, not sure for a moment if I was still pregnant.

I wasn't. But I also was—there was a dead embryo inside me. I needed to stop feeling pregnant.

I had my morning cry, made breakfast, then placed the two pills under my tongue and let them dissolve.

I talked to my body while I waited for the pills to work their way through my system. We were going to have to go through this together.

I'm sorry. This is going to be hard and it's going to hurt. I'm sorry we have to go through this. But I will take care of you.

I hadn't had any connection to my body since I was seven years old. I'd made it the villain of my life story—I blamed everything on it. If I didn't get the part, I blamed my body. If I didn't get the guy, I blamed my body. If I didn't like who I was, I blamed my body. But I didn't want to blame it anymore. I wanted a truce. I wasn't ready to love it, but I didn't want to hate it anymore.

ENDING AN ERA

I was counting down the days until we could start trying again. I wanted to pretend like none of it had ever happened. Soomsoom would just be a blip in our lives that we'd forget once there was a *Pereg* ("poppy seed") or *Boten* ("peanut") to dote on.

I'd never put much stock in the five-stages-of-grief idea. People in my life had died, and I'd been sad and missed them, but I always understood and accepted it. Miscarrying was something else. I couldn't justify it. I knew that miscarriages were common. I knew that it didn't mean I'd never have another baby. I knew that Soomsoom hadn't had any thoughts or feelings—he wasn't a person who had died tragically; he wasn't even a he yet. I wasn't mourning a baby that I'd held in my arms and cared for and loved. I didn't miss him; I didn't know him (or her). I understood that I was mourning the idea that I was going to be a mother, the experience of being pregnant. I just needed to get over it and do it again. Denial was a really nice phase.

Anger was less nice. I'd never been particularly good at anger. I'd cry when I was angry. I'd get quiet when I was angry, shut off and keep it inside me, until I managed to convince myself that it was an unnecessary emotion altogether; it doesn't serve a purpose, and it just makes things worse, so just let it go, and if it won't go, then tuck it away.

I would have done that, but the anger snuck up on me. It was a hot summer night, and I was ten different kinds of exhausted, and I'd had two glasses of pinot grigio with dinner. Roy left to walk Inez, and the apartment was quiet, except for the swirling of the ceiling fan. I lay back on the couch and stared at it. Then I got angry, all of a sudden and overwhelmingly. Tears started pouring out of me, soaking the throw pillow beneath my head. I cried, increasingly loud and hard. I thought it might make me feel better to curse—I remembered stubbing my toe in the backyard as a kid and looking at my mom for permission to say a bad word, and she nodded and said, "Sometimes cursing makes it feel a little bit better"—so I cursed. Out loud. At the fan. Like a crazy person.

"Fuck you, you asshole! Fuck you!!"

It wasn't the fan's fault that I had miscarried, but it was directly above me and it'd do. It wasn't the fan I was cursing at anyway.

I've never been a religious person. Even as a kid, God and religion were separate ideas in my mind; religion was a culture, a history I had some place in. God was something I didn't understand but needed to believe existed because there needed to be a reason why so much of my life had been so hard. Everything that's happened in my life—growing up in garbage with rats and homeless people living in my home, my house burning down when I was seven, my mother's series of surgeries that almost killed her, even my constant struggle with my own body—there had to have been a purpose to it all. Maybe it was to make me stronger, or to make me kinder and more empathetic, who knows. But what reason could there be for me to lose my baby?

"I've hit my quota, do you hear me? No more. I can't handle any more. Either kill me or give me a fucking break. Do you hear me?" I screamed. "Do you fucking hear me?!"

"I hear you, and so do our neighbors." Roy was home.

Inez immediately found a spot under the bed to hide from me. She hadn't gone near me since the miscarriage. I thought it was the scent of the blood, but it could have been that I was losing my mind.

"I'm always here with you," he told me. "You don't have to go through any of this alone."

"Yes, I do. You can't bleed out our baby." I was going on eleven straight days of bleeding. The embryo was already gone, but the blood kept coming. "I have to do that by myself. So take your comforting words and your helpless looks and leave me alone."

He did, letting me cry myself to sleep on the couch. He woke up early the next morning to walk the dog and let me sleep off my embarrassment.

I said I was sorry, and he said not to be, that I didn't need to be. That he understood. "Your life hasn't been easy, babe." There was a lecture coming. "But you grew up a middle-class white girl in the northeastern United States. As far as shitty lives go, the majority of the world has it worse than you."

"I know," I said.

"There are kids who don't even wipe the flies off their eyeballs. "

"I know."

"ISIS is kidnapping and selling children as sex slaves."

"I know. I'm sorry," I said. "I feel stupid. I guess I'm a little angry."

He brought me a glass of water and stroked my hair. "You can be angry. I am. But you need to keep it proportional."

"I don't know how to keep it proportional," I said. "In the grand scheme it's not a big deal, right? It happens all the time. Miscarrying is not the worst thing that's ever happened to me. I don't know why I can't stop being so sad."

"Because it's sad," he said. "I don't think the sadness is going to go away until you're pregnant again. But you can't let it take over."

"Let's just get pregnant again."

"Ready when you are," he said.

I thought I was ready. I bided my time until the doctor said we could try again by learning everything I could about my system. I did all the things I said I didn't want to do, like buying ovulation kits and taking my temperature first thing every morning. But when the two months had passed and we'd finally been given the green light to make a new baby, I wasn't as sure as I thought I was.

For years I'd treated my body like a project on my to-do list. I simply needed to research and put in the work, and then it would be fixed, and I could move on to the next thing. Except there was never a next thing—I always had this body. But the ongoing physical and emotional trauma of bleeding out my dead baby for an entire month forced me to communicate with my body in a way other than expecting it to behave a certain way and getting frustrated when it didn't. Being attentive to it and worrying about its well-being did more to connect me to my body than all the years of diets and workouts and research and writing about health and fitness had ever done. It wasn't a happy ending; it wasn't even a silver lining. I wished desperately that I'd never been pregnant at all, but I had been, and now I was in a lot of pain, every day. So I focused on keeping my promise to my body that I'd take care of it.

"I think you're right," I told Roy while we sat on the couch prepping Netflix. "I think we should wait until I get healthier to have a baby."

"When did I say that?"

"When we were talking about getting pregnant."

"Kim, you can't just randomly continue conversations that happened months ago and think that I'm going to understand what's happening."

"Sorry, it's been on my mind."

"I don't think we have to stop trying; we can lose weight while we try." Always "we" when weight was the topic.

"It's not just the weight. I need to be in a better place with myself."

He pulled me in for a kiss on the head and squeezed me tight, then pressed play on an episode of *Unbreakable Kimmy Schmidt*.

I lost six pounds the week after my miscarriage, two pounds the week after that, then two more and two more. Losing weight was becoming infuriatingly easy. I no longer needed to take a nap to get through the day. My concentration was better. Itchy patches of dry skin that I'd had for years cleared up virtually overnight. Besides an underlying sadness in everything I did and a compulsive need to avoid pregnant women, I felt better than I had in at least a decade. My body was finally functioning properly. It was the hormones my endocrinologist had prescribed, the hormones that I'd needed to stay pregnant. When I asked him why no one had thought to give me Synthroid sooner, he suggested that I just be happy we'd caught it when we did.

I needed a little more time with my body, alone, to be selfish, to find some balance, to reincorporate my body into my sense of self. It sounded like some hippie-dippy, lovey-dovey blog I'd write for a women's magazine, but I'd spent a large part of my life as an out-of-body experience. I'd had years of excuses why I couldn't just let myself be normal, but I wasn't acting anymore; I wasn't on stage or on camera, and no one called me regularly for my measurements. I wasn't a dancer anymore. The only diet pills I would be taking from here on out were the ones I needed to regulate my thyroid. There were no more pageants in my future. I wasn't trying to keep an ex from cheating or trying to win Roy with my commitment to starvation. There was no more wedding day to diet for. How I felt about my body was dictated by what society had told me that I should feel, depending on how I conformed to its norms. But there was no more external pressure to pin it on; it was just me. It didn't go away—the standard was still a size two—but I stopped caring so much about how I thought others thought I looked. I was the one unhappy with the way I looked, and I was the one I was answerable to.

Even if I never lost another pound, I needed to reach peace with myself. The only pictures I had with my mother were from my wedding. I didn't want to be the kind of mom who never took pictures with her family. Didn't leave memories for her children to hold on to. I didn't want to pass on my deep-seated insecurities to my kids: they tend to pick up everything, and I didn't want them growing up thinking that was normal and okay.

Even if I was genetically suited for the Ice Age, even if there were obese people in the Paleolithic era and people had been dieting since the dawn of civilization, it was all just information. It didn't change my life in any way (well, maybe a little in winter). It's what we do at the end of the day, not what we think, that matters. So I decided to fake it, to start treating my body like it belonged to someone I loved.

I looked in the mirror, really looked, at everything about me that I'd always looked away from. I had to admit to myself that I was not the person I thought I was. I wasn't the size six I was when I tried to win my husband, but I wasn't the monster I'd created in my mind. I was overweight. Worse things had happened to me than buying bigger pants.

I started making a list of all the things I needed to do to learn to be happy with my body: throw away my scale, cut all the tags out of my clothes, leave affirmations of self-love on my bathroom mirror. I would do all the things that I'd always said I'd do when I was thin enough, like taking trapeze lessons and boudoir photo shoots and wearing a bikini. It was the kind of list I'd write for work, and when I was done reading it over, I deleted it. My body wasn't on my to-do list anymore. I needed to actually take some time to live in it the way it was instead of hiding from it.

I started taking pictures with Roy again—I would no longer pretend that this period in my life never happened. It was part of my journey. I started dressing like I liked getting dressed. I'd spent the last two years in search of the most nondescript clothing I could find, loose, neutral tops and cardigans meant to distract from my width. I didn't want to be noticed; I wanted to blend into the background. I was losing weight through no real fault of my own, but I wasn't going to delude myself into thinking I'd end up as thin as I'd been when I ate seven hundred calories and exercised two hours a day. I was going to let my body find a new normal, some balance I could live in that wouldn't require me to focus all my time and energy on maintaining. Since I didn't know what size I'd end up as, I decided not to buy a whole new wardrobe; I subscribed to a wardrobe-rental website, where I could pick out a few outfits each month and wear them for as long as I wanted and then return them for something new. I had clothes that were nice, that fit me, and I didn't need to feel uncomfortable in the dressing room of Banana Republic.

I'd spent years dedicated to fitness trends, doing exercises and workouts that I hated but knew would change my life. I quit them. I decided to just do the things that I enjoyed, even if they weren't perfect, supereffective routines. It was okay. I would move and do something healthy, even if it didn't burn the exact same number of calories I allowed myself to eat that day.

I stopped reading the fitness magazines I'd religiously consumed and had aspired to run one day. They never said anything new anyway.

There are seven billion bodies in the world, and I got this one. It may not be the best one, but it's far from being the worst. It comes from a long line of people who have survived things much more harrowing than social-media bullying or miscarriages. I've gotten the best they had to offer. It's a strong body and a soft body, and while it's not as beautiful as I'd have liked, it's the only one I will ever have, so I'm working on being thankful for it. I will always love diets and the hope they give me, but I will love them for what they are, a fantasy, and I will not let them hurt me again. Chasing the ideal body is like chasing the horizon—it's all a matter of perspective. I'll never really get there, but I'll appreciate the view as I try.

EPILOGUE

"Do you want to sit down?" A woman about my mother's age is tugging on my coat, already starting to stand.

"No, I'm fine. But thank you," I tell her. "I'm only going a couple of stops."

I've been offered seats before over the years, a combination of big coats, weight gain, and bad posture at the end of the workday. Those well-meant offers haunted me. Sent me spiraling into a depression that always resulted in some form of punishment involving more cardio and fewer carbs. And that instinct is still there. To question my body and how it's betrayed me this time, but I shake it off.

I look over at Roy, and he's grinning from ear to ear. "You look pregnant."

"I know," I say.

In the past twenty-two weeks I've gained seven pounds, but it looks like more. My face has thinned, but my breasts are huge, and the roundness of my belly has moved up and up and up. I have officially had to transition out of pants that button, and my maternity jeans have just started to reach the point where I don't have to pull them up constantly. I look pregnant.

There are some habits that die hard, and each month on my way to the doctor, I make sure whatever it is I'm wearing is on the light side. I pee first, and as I step on the scale I make a mental note of my start weight. I can't help but look at the nurse for reassurance, that I haven't gained too much and at the same time that I've gained enough.

It doesn't seem to matter what I do; my body does what it wants these days, and I have happily taken my hands off the wheel. I'd been so careful before, last time, making sure I got the exact number of macronutrients recommended by my *Eating Well When You're Expecting* book, choosing all my food from an approved list of baby-body-and-brain-boosting foods. I wanted to be perfectly pregnant.

This time I'm really into beef, pickles, and halibut—oh, halibut, where have you been all my life? Broccoli is gross, but I can eat carrots by the bushel. And milk. My god how I love milk, the kind with the fat in it that I never allowed myself to drink before.

I'm so hungry. All the time, I'm hungry. I like it. I've never been this hungry before and it's great. I wonder if this is what normal people feel like; in tune with the fact that their body wants something and so very willing to give in to its demands even if that means getting up from bed in the middle of the night for a snack.

I know it won't always be like this, but I hope it will. Not the hungry part, the being okay with being hungry part. The eating when I need it part and seeing food as a sum of its parts, not just as a number of calories to be deducted from my daily allowance. For the first time in my life eating isn't hard. It's not emotional. It's just a sandwich.

The Internet told me that it would be harder this time, to relax, to enjoy being pregnant. After a loss, the anonymous masses said, I would worry about everything and have a harder time connecting to my pregnancy.

Today is Soomsoom's due date, and as we get off the subway en route to visit friends with a new baby of their own, I wish him a happy birthday in my head. I will always know how old he or she would be. But I'm okay. The Internet was wrong. I'm not worried; I knew from the moment that the line turned pink that this little guy was okay. And that I was okay. And that I was hungry.

ACKNOWLEDGMENTS

Vivian Lee, my editor. Thank you. This was such a journey, and while I know this book (and its author) landed on your lap out of nowhere, you handled this process with such grace, patience, and talent. Thank you for your unfailing support and guidance.

To my agent, Mollie Glick, thank you for always being my champion, cheerleader, and bad guy.

Dennelle Catlett, my fairy godpublicist. My love for you borders on awkward. I'm owning it. You are wonderful.

Mom and Dad, I promise to not write anything else about you. You're off the hook. I love you bigger than the world.

Roy Schwartz, you're still my happy ending. Always. I hope to one day be as good at life as you think I am. Thank you for your overnight edits, early-morning dog walks, and limitless support; I can't remember how I did life before you.

Ethan Dean Schwartz, as I write this you are mere days away from leaving this body of mine and entering the world, with all its joy and judgment. I don't know yet the color of your hair or eyes, whether you've inherited my cleft chin or your father's square jaw, whether you'll be tall or small or broad or narrow. My only hope for your body is that you love it. Appreciate all the generations who survived to pass on each curve and quirk that makes you perfectly, beautifully you. Making you is the most amazing thing this body of mine has ever done.

SELECTED BIBLIOGRAPHY

Primary Text

Banner, Lois W. *American Beauty: A Social History . . . Through Two Centuries of the American Idea, Ideal, and Image of the Beautiful Woman.* Los Angeles: Figueroa Press, 2005.

Bourlière, François, and Clark F. Howell, eds. *African Ecology and Human Evolution.* London, New York: Routledge, 2013 (reprint, original printing 1964).

Brumberg, Joan Jacobs. *The Body Project: An Intimate History of American Girls.* New York: Random House, 1997.

Carson, Gerald. *Cornflake Crusade.* New York: Rinehart & Company, 1957.

Etcoff, Nancy. *Survival of the Prettiest: The Science of Beauty.* New York: Random House, 1999.

Foxcroft, Louise. *Calories and Corsets: A History of Dieting over 2,000 Years.* London: Profile Books, 2012.

Kolata, Gina. *Rethinking Thin: The New Science of Weight Loss—and the Myths and Realities of Dieting.* New York: Picador, 2008.

Lieberman, Daniel E. *The Story of the Human Body: Evolution, Health, and Disease*. New York: Random House, 2013.

Nissenbaum, Stephen. *Sex, Diet, and Debility in Jacksonian America*. Westport, CT: Greenwood Press, 1980.

Panati, Charles. *The Browser's Book of Endings*. New York: Penguin Books, 1999. (Originally published as *Panati's Extraordinary Endings of Practically Everything and Everybody* by Perennial Library, 1989.)

Russell, Phillips. *William the Conqueror*. New York: Charles Scribner's Sons, 1933.

Schwartz, Hillel. *Never Satisfied: A Cultural History of Diets, Fantasies and Fat*. New York: The Free Press (Macmillan, Inc.), 1986.

Vigarello, Georges. *The Metamorphoses of Fat: A History of Obesity*. New York: Columbia University Press, 2013.

Yager, Susan. *The Hundred Year Diet: America's Voracious Appetite for Losing Weight*. New York: Rodale, 2010.

Zee, Henri A. van der. *The Hunger Winter: Occupied Holland 1944–1945*. London: Jill Norman & Hobhouse, 1982.

Journals and Reports

Ashwell, M., P. Gunn, and S. Gibson. "Waist-to-Height Ratio Is a Better Screening Tool Than Waist Circumference and BMI for Adult Cardiometabolic Risk Factors: Systematic Review and Meta-analysis." *Obesity Reviews* 13, no. 3 (2011): 275–86. doi:10.1111/j.1467-789X.2011.00952.x.

Burley, Nancy. "Sexual Selection for Aesthetic Traits in Species with Biparental Care." *The American Naturalist* 127, no. 4 (1986): 415–45. Print. doi:10.1086/284493.

Byars, Sean G., Douglas Ewbank, Govindaraju R. Diddahally, and Stephen C. Stearns. "Natural Selection in a Contemporary Human Population." *Proceedings of the National Academy of Sciences* 107, suppl. 1 (2009): 1787–792. Print. doi:10.1073/pnas.0906199106.

Dixson, Alan F., and Barnaby J. Dixson. "Venus Figurines of the European Paleolithic: Symbols of Fertility or Attractiveness?" *Journal of Anthropology* 2011 (2011): 11 pages. Web. doi:10.1155/2011/569120.

Flegal, K. M., B. K. Kit, H. Orpana, and B. I. Graubard. "Association of All-Cause Mortality with Overweight and Obesity Using Standard Body Mass Index Categories: A Systematic Review and Meta-analysis." *JAMA* 309, no. 1 (2013): 71–82. doi:10.1001/jama.2012.113905.

Hacker, David J. "Decennial Life Tables for the White Population of the United States, 1790–1900." *Historical Methods: A Journal of Quantitative and Interdisciplinary History* 43, no. 2 (2010): 45–79. Web. doi:10.1080/01615441003720449.

Hart, Nicky. "Famine, Maternal Nutrition and Infant Mortality: A Re-Examination of the Dutch Hunger Winter." *Population Studies* 47, no. 1 (1993): 27–46. Print. doi:10.1080/0032472031000146716.

Kalm, Leah M., and Richard D. Semba. "They Starved So That Others Be Better Fed: Remembering Ancel Keys and the Minnesota Experiment." *The American Society for Nutritional Sciences* 135, no. 6 (2005): 1347–352. Print.

Karremans, Johan C., Willem E. Frankenhuis, and Sander Arons. "Blind Men Prefer a Low Waist-to-Hip Ratio." *Evolution and Human Behavior* 31, no. 3 (2010): 182–86. doi:10.1016/j.evolhumbehav.2009.10.001.

Lassek, William D., and Steven J. C. Gaulin. "Waist-Hip Ratio and Cognitive Ability: Is Gluteofemoral Fat a Privileged Store of Neurodevelopmental Resources?" *Evolution and Human Behavior* 29, no. 1 (2008): 26–34. doi:10.1016/j.evolhumbehav.2007.07.005.

Pai, Seeta, and Kelly Schryver. "Children, Teens, Media, and Body Image: A Common Sense Media Research Brief." San Francisco: Common Sense Media. 2015.

Prum, Richard O. "Aesthetic Evolution by Mate Choice: Darwin's Really Dangerous Idea." *Philosophical Transactions of the Royal Society B: Biological Sciences* 367, no. 1600 (2012): 2253–265. Web. Accessed 11 May 2016. doi:10.1098/rstb.2011.0285.

Ruff, Christopher B. "Climate and Body Shape in Hominid Evolution." *Journal of Human Evolution* 21, no. 2 (1991): 81–105. Print. doi:10.1016/0047-2484(91)90001-c.

Schlebusch, C.M., et al. "Genomic Variation in Seven Khoe-San Groups Reveals Adaptation and Complex African History." *Science* 338, no. 6105 (2012): 374–79. doi:10.1126/science.1227721.

Schulz, Laura. "The Dutch Hunger Winter and the Developmental Origins of Health and Disease." *Proceedings of the National Academy of Sciences* 107, no. 39 (2010): 16757–6758. Print. doi:10.1073/pnas.1012911107.

Singh, D. "Adaptive Significance of Female Physical Attractiveness: Role of Waist-to-Hip Ratio." *Journal of Personality and Social Psychology* 65, no. 2 (1993): 293–307. doi:10.1037//0022-3514.65.2.293.

Singh, D. "Ideal Female Body Shape: Role of Body Weight and Waist-to-Hip Ratio." *International Journal of Eating Disorders* 16, no. 3 (1994): 283–88. doi:10.1002/1098-108x(199411)16:33.0.co;2-q.

Singh, D. "Universal Allure of the Hourglass Figure: An Evolutionary Theory of Female Physical Attractiveness." *Clinics in Plastic Surgery* 33, no. 3 (2006): 359–70. doi:10.1016/j.cps.2006.05.007.

Spalding, Kirsty, et al. "Dynamics of Fat Cell Turnover in Humans." *Nature* 453 (June 2008): 783-787. Print. doi:10.1038/nature06902.

Stulp, Gert, Louise Barrett, Felix C. Tropf, and Melinda Mills. "Does Natural Selection Favour Taller Stature Among the Tallest People on Earth?" *Proceedings of the Royal Society B: Biological Sciences* 282, no. 1806 (2015): 2015–211. doi:10.1098/rspb.2015.0211.

Sutin, Angelina R., and Antonio Terracciano. "Body Weight Misperception in Adolescence and Incident Obesity in Young Adulthood." *Psychological Science* 26, no. 4 (2015): 507–11. Print. doi:10.1177/0956797614566319.

Articles

Bergner, Daniel. "The Anatomy of Desire." *New York Times*, April 16, 2010.

Gadsby, Patricia, and Leon Steele. "The Inuit Paradox: How Can People Who Gorge on Fat and Rarely See a Vegetable Be Healthier Than We Are?" *Discover*, October 1, 2004.

Khan, Razib. "The Bushmen Tell Us a Lot about Human Evolution Because They Are Humans Who Have Evolved." *Discover*, September 21, 2012.

University of the Witwatersrand. "Khoe-San Peoples Diverged Before 'Out-of-Africa' Migration of Modern Humans." ScienceDaily, September 20, 2012. http://www.sciencedaily.com /releases/2012/09/120920141139.htm.

Zimmer, Carl. "Natural Selection May Help Account for Dutch Height Advantage." *New York Times*, April 9, 2015.

Photos

The Battle Creek Sanitarium. The New York Public Library Digital Collections, Rare Book Division, the New York Public Library, New York. Accessed May 13, 2016. http://digitalcollections.nypl .org/items/c37c22b3-2577-835e-e040-e00a18066b39.

Battle Creek Sanitarium Health Foods. The New York Public Library Art and Picture Collection, the New York Public Library Digital Collections, New York. Accessed May 13, 2016. http:// digitalcollections.nypl.org/items/510d47e1-38d3-a3d9-e040 -e00a18064a99.

INDEX

ABOUT THE AUTHOR

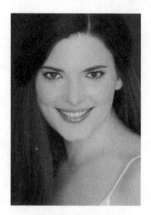

Photo © Chris Macke

Kimberly Rae Miller is a bestselling author, editor, and blogger. Her 2013 memoir, *Coming Clean*, was picked by both Amazon and *Elle* magazine as one of the best books of the year, and it was a nominee for the 2013 Goodreads Choice Awards. She has written on healthy living for numerous magazines and websites, including her personal blog, www.TheKimChallenge.com. Kim lives in New York City.